Call it MS – My Story

Multiple Sclerosis takes My Senses but not My Soul

First Edition. V.03

Written by Adrian A C Johnson

ISBN 978-1-365-10985-0

www.CallItMS.com

ISBN 978-1-365-10985-0

Legal

Dedication

My Source of inspiration is My Saviour. He washed My Soul and lifted My Spirit to this place where I can share My Story with earnest recollect and touch the hearts of those who turn these pages. I have been blessed with the true love of friends and family which makes it impossible to single out anyone earthly. None of their love would have been possible without the smallest touch of the Almighty. These words compiled here are all the influence of Our Father who guides my pen, fingers and mind. Our Father raised me up from my darkest moment and lit the way that I might travel and share the moments with you.

I thank Our Father for all He has done to make it possible for me to share this story and praise His holiness that He afforded me friends and family like you who have encouraged me even in the smallest way to live.

Preface

The following is a compilation of some of the Moments Shared leading up to and following my diagnosis with Multiple Sclerosis (MS). It is not a chronology or journal, just memories caught or triggered by the day to day happenings, these years later.

References are made to technical matters that may not be accurate. They are only my perceptions and I do not purport to be technically minded in any of the matters referred to herein. This compilation is my perspective and true expressions of my heart with no desire to mislead. I apologize for any misunderstanding I may have caused and hope that you appreciate these words, though conveyed in earnest, are delivered by an imperfect man who seeks the graces of our Lord and Savior.

Acknowledgement

Had not for the insistence of friends, both in person and on social media, I would not have attempted to compile the brief stories of my life into book form. I wish to thank you all for the encouragement and hope that these words bring some desired clarity, pleasure and inspiration.

Author's Profile

The author is the third of four children born to parents Adrian and Mavine Johnson of Barbados. Adrian Johnson Jr. became diagnosed with Multiple Sclerosis in 2005 and has been battling the illness since then. His writing started in 2014 after sharing some of his story in post on social media.

Adrian was a retail Manager with the largest Regional Stationery and later, after a brief Management role with the retailing arms of Starcom Network, returned to Brydens before retiring ill.

CONTENTS	Page

Some of you

Like some of you, I passed them too and gave them a dollar. In fact, I dug deep into my pockets and shared, when I thought their requests were legitimate, but that left me to judge their circumstances. It was good to help where and when I could. But what if I said no to someone whose beseeching was unconvincing? What if I made a cursory judgment, like some of you may have done too and walked away.

Too many of our brothers and sisters fall on bad luck and become destitute. Regrettably far too many roam our towns and their allies, streets and their corners, and just about everywhere else, wearing sheep's clothing. Pretending they are who they are not, in hopes of charming the generous and humane quality in you or appealing to your empathy to solicit money and feed their addictions or greed. There was a documentary featuring the street beggars who in reality were career beggars, some having substantial means to go home to. Some went as far as to pretend disabilities, so as to convince more readily. They used props like wheelchairs, crutches, eye patches, walking sticks, dark shades and more.

To take someone's property by deception is stealing, if it isn't legally theft, it ought to be. Con Men Should be arrested and jailed for their deceptions when caught. For me it is a worse crime, this theft by deception, playing on people's emotions to swindle them out of their dollars. But in our society, deception seems to have become such a norm, merchants capitalize on their abilities to deceive. Ads are deliberately fashioned to exploit and bleed even your last dollar. There is little respect for another person's hard earned money and professionals seek to get unscrupulous shares of it. Industries design ways to have you coming back and there are even industries specifically targeting the sick. Man's morality has stooped so low in some of our brothers and sisters, to say they use gutter practices is to elevate them beyond their realistic stratum. The serpent may have crawled the earth but his glory was from the pits of hell. Deception of any kind is a cruelty, when we deceive the emotions and hopes of others, we crawl with serpents and sleep in their dens.

For many of us it is harder to be truthful than it is to lie. Unfortunately truth has become a stranger, dressed beyond recognition. Even when it stares us in the face, we are so guarded from being deceived, we turn away with our new found ease,

living in a fraudulent maxim, "He's too honest to be trusted!"

These last ten years I have spent at home away from society, most of my time

sitting semi clothed, having no visitors and seeing no fresh faces. My only trips

were to the doctors, clinics or labs. I had a handful of outings in this time that

were not medically related and three were funerals where I paid my sincere

condolences and left without conversation. For years I couldn't see the screen to

use the computer and when my eyes started to perceive color again, the muscles

were so unaccustomed to sight, the screen would pulse, in and out after spending

fifteen minutes at it. There were no windows to the outside world accessible but

four years ago, the pulsing steadied to a much weaker tremor and I could endure

hours at a time. The computer became my window and with the help of a friend in

France and another who was combing the globe, I set up a Facebook account and so

the window opened into your homes and hearts. In somewhat naivety, I trusted

that what you saw looking back would have been my honest day to day life and not

some deception. I am properly informed about the scamming and trickery in the brave new world of the Internet and its social media but somehow I was misguided. I believed my nakedness was apparent and that there was no likelihood of being discerned for a sheep and in the absence of fangs, no chance of being called a wolf, cunning with deception. Truth is a stranger even with this microscopic focus. I was jarred to this reality when I published and learned the thirty hours I spent over this last weekend getting the book published, were also unrecognized, some believe the book was in motion long ago.

Each chapter was written the day it was posted, as is this chapter. I included them as I will this but there is no cloak to remove, my heart is revealed and My Spirit trusts with injury. I will renew My Strength as My Sustenance is from an eternal source. I published them in reverse order, the most recent being the first and there is no sequence to my memories. It is not a chronology of my illness or a journal of my life but rather it is my raw recollection of passed moments triggered by present circumstances. The choice to use an editor to make the text more grammatically correct and easier to read was one I declined. I would not have had the same literary manipulation, had you been sitting here in the living room with me. My posts were invitations to have your right here, honest dissertations of thoughts that would never serve for dialogue in a face to face visit but monologues that beckon your ear.

There is no cloak and dagger, no testing of waters to measure its depth. I took the risk of openness but it was never risky. I have not yet learned the ease of lies, those I told in an imperfect past, took great effort from me and are more difficult to maintain. This sedentary life has given me the kind of opportunity I never availed myself of before. I now have the time to smell the roses and when I next walk through rows of their bushes or pass gardens on my way to scheduled meets, I will stop and smell them. Until then, I savor the blessings that unveil as I open My Screen to reveal your kind friendliness. As my friend from my roots in Deacons road and alma mater said to me, "Deacons road boys do not give up. Up and on my friend."

Road Blocks

When they told me my mother would be leaving for England, I understood. My first day at school when she left, I sat quietly but the boy next to Me Screamed and was inconsolable. It must have been from watching her leave for work and returning in the evening that had prepared me for the waves bye-bye. And when she and my dad left at night for their infrequent trips to the cinema, I understood and didn't cry then either. So this trip to England when I was five, was understood, at least as far as a child that age should be expected to. What I didn't understand was that it was late evening and she didn't return. I woke in the morning and ran to her room, but she wasn't there.

When I finally got used to the idea, I looked forward to her returning still but more bravely, knowing that a letter was to first come and inform us the date. I ran to the mailman whenever I heard the motorcycle but the wait was like an eternity, although my mom wrote regularly. One of the things that grabbed me about her letters was the way she formed the letter "M" in her name. I loved it so much, I tried to copy it and when nearing perfection, I decided to learn to write some other letters in her style, it made me feel closer to her.

The M in her name became like a landmark of achievement, I copied it better than the other letters. My handwriting improved tremendously and soon gained me an award for penmanship. I represented My School in an island wide competition but placed miserably when on competition day, my dad got me there thirty minutes after it started and my haste to finish left a dismal distortion of my celebrated handwriting. The memory of an imperfect capital "S" haunted me and many years afterwards, My Scribbled "S," became an awkward trademark. I still made a very legible "M" but my "S" was sometimes flat headed and other times, big bellied. I had some trouble with my "E" too, it was so irregular, often top heavy or big footed, but it was never as significant, since I used comparatively fewer "Es" in my opening sentences.

These two letters may have been speaking to me all my life. My mother's initials were MS when she was carrying me the first eight months. I went to her wedding and was a December gift for her one month later. My Steady girlfriend at school was also initialed MS and because of the age difference, her wisdom positively influenced all my following relationships. When the doctor told me MS, my mind was not cast on these memories, I could think of nothing other than the life change that was looming. The more I think of MS now, the more I feel to make Mock Sport of these haunting letters. The "M's" in my life that brought inspiration and influenced me to be better, like my mom and sweetheart. The "S's" that destroyed my penmanship and was discarded by these females in marriage. MS has brought many good things in my life along with the devastation. MS – My Soul, My Strength, My Spirit, My Savior, all things that now make Me Safe from the destruction of My Senses.

Multiple Sclerosis (MS) is an autoimmune disease and is therefore related to others like Lupus and myasthenia gravis (MG). In this family of diseases, the immune system is believed to run rogue and it attacks healthy body cells. In Lupus, it's the organ tissue and skin, in MG it's the muscles and in this dreaded MS, the nerves. The nerves are responsible for carrying impulses to and responses back from the Central Nervous System (CNS). They do so electrically. The CNS comprises the Brain, Optic Nerves in the eyes, the Spinal Cord and the millions of nerves in a Network running throughout the body. The impulses and responses are conveyed as messages through the complex network of nerves, leaping from one to the next, all the way to the brain for interpretation and back. This passing of information has to be perfectly transmitted, from the moment an impulse is triggered at the nerves' receptors. The impulse travels by leaping from nerve to nerve, passing through high end traffic at better than lightning speeds, without colliding and reaching the brain uncorrupted. The doctors may test the soles of the feet during investigation to see if the sensation of soft touch is confused with needle pricks, to judge the condition of ones nerves. You may remember the pinching of toes when a person had been in a crippling accident or was unconscious for a period of time. Again, it is the investigation of impulses reaching the brain and the healthy function of nerves. The nerves are More Sensitive than any man made scaling device as is evident in the sensitive facial nerves that can detect the lightest touch of a fly's wing, yet they interpret the distinct difference of a kiss from a slap.

Nerves are likened to electrical wires. It is a crude comparison of these wondrously made cells to man's poor attempts at sending impulses. Nonetheless, the outer sheath of insulation on a wire serves to protect inner strands, and allow functionality. Breakage in this insulating sheath will result in interrupted flow of the electricity. The nerve has a similar outer sheath made of fatty lipids, called myelin. Myelin protects the integrity of its inner strands. It is in fact the destruction of this myelin layer by the immune system that causes the malfunctioning of nerves throughout the body, a road block of sorts. Like electrical wires, the damaged nerves will have breakages in communication throughout the CNS which are manifested as the symptoms in multiple sclerosis like trouble walking, muscle weakness or spasms, blurred or double vision, numbness and tingling and more tragic ones, perhaps too depressing to visit.

These academic symptoms do not include manifestations so agonizing they redefine MS. Nerves control the memory centre and your perception. The memory of every moment you've lived, good or bad, is stored and although you don't readily recall them all, stimulation can cause the resurfacing of these memories. The doctors didn't warn you, nor did literature. The flashes of previous knife attacks can surface as real as the very night. Or the dog bite when you were only five years, feels as harsh as when it first bled. In fact, if you look at the leg, you Might See the blood dripping. Confused nerve messages can be so corrupted, tragedies long behind you can replay with equal horridness. Phantom impulses can be so convincing, the fire from your childhood seems to burn with equal intensity.

MS - is only Mock Sport to me because the ghost impulses I experience, are actually confused Messages Spreading throughout. Remember that experiment of whispering a message across the room from person to person and discovering that "Meet me in the back later" is corrupted so badly it could become as twisted as "Sweet potato on a cracked platter." When we hear the end message, we often laugh at the metamorphosis of the spoken word. Well, a gentle touch can now pierce My Skin like a dagger and a slap can be More Soothing.

The simple letters M and S have now evolved so significantly in my life, I highlight them with capitals often when they fall in side by side words, as a reminder that although this debilitating illness thrives to overcome My Senses, I have grown

More Spiritual and it will not take My Soul.

Capping – Partial decapitation

When he raised the blade over his captor's pinky finger and heard him begging, "Please don't!" his responding threat was "You are going to beg to have me cut it off!" I smiled because my thoughts were, is he kidding, how on earth could he expect someone to beg to have their finger removed. My naivety of torturing skills had shielded me from a cruel world but I was rudely awakened with agonizing screams of "Cut it off, please, cut it off!" echoing inwardly as I shared his agony. The movie was so realistic, I felt myself slipping into the scene and being the captive. Pain had become resident in me and when I saw others in pain, they became like family, sharing my roof. Even this fictitious screen character, a man deserving of some payback for his atrocities, didn't deserve this excruciating pain and he received my empathy.

Our bodies are made up with an incredible self-healing nature, once our cells are allowed to function naturally, they mend almost every conceivable ill. We all have cancer daily to unnoticeable degrees. If we accept cancer to be the amassing of cells into growing clusters, then regular phagocytic behavior of white blood cells, engulfing and absorbing harmful microorganisms or any dangerous foreign bodies, in growing cluster, is cancer. There is a school of thought, I am obviously a sympathizer, which believes cancer is when this natural clearing activity runs amuck due largely to an imbalance of internal status. With increased acidity in the body, cells behave inefficiently and can seldom carryout maximal functionality. The more acidic we are, the more likely the phagocytes will blunder and the clusters grow out of control into a dangerous tumors.

As informed as I thought I was, my ignorance to the workings of the blood clot medication Warfin was verified. I was of the impression that once I took this rat poison, it would eat away at the blood clot, and dwindle it to nothingness. A more enlightened mind now understands that the blood thinner attempts to render the blood to a healthier status and allow the cells to do unimpeded work. The white blood cells when they encounter a blockage, like miners in a blocked tunnel after a cave in, take away small bits and redeposit them for elimination on functioning tracks.

My blood clot was still in the process of being dismantled and my regular intake of Warfin was to ensure the cells' work was continuous. While they carried out their work, I tried to adapt to a new state of life. I knew car rides were going to be painful but I needed my regular trips to the doctors. I mapped out that the pain was greatest during rapid wheel turns and vibrations, like the swerving to avoid collisions and potholes. Initially I thought it was going into the potholes that brought the severe discomfort. As much as that shook me up, the rapid tug to avoid them was worse. My dad was the best person to drive me although admittedly, and I hope I don't damage our gender pride, my mom was always the better driver. He drove in the middle of the road where there were fewer irregularities on its surface and therefore, had no need to swerve off of potholes and seldom went through any. Due to his sluggish speed, there were seldom sudden brakes.

With seniority of driving years and being head of the family, he always took the wheel when we had an outing. To see My Sister off at the airport was going to be my only outing, other than on medical related trips. We were concerned given the distance but it was a family tradition I didn't want to break and I prepared to deal with this dragon. One reassurance was that the road to the airport was smooth highway. I felt a bit disoriented when we got there but my Motion Sickness was quick to leave after some rest. The trip back was a different beast. My dad missed the lane to the highway and went the coast road. The sensations were new and if we had been previously introduced, I would have broken tradition for fear of meeting them again.

I describe it as "Capping" because it felt like a cap on my head and its band was getting tighter with each motion of the wheel, turns or vibrations. When I appealed with agony, my mom asked if we should stop. That was my "Cut it off" moment. I felt like I would have them partially decapitate me. I wanted to be out of the car but I needed to get home for my medication. I told them to drive and braced myself on the dashboard with both hands but that only augmented the vibrations. There was no taming this dragon, it burned its fury through me and at the end of the trip, when we finally got home, I was crisp, brittle and falling to pieces. Ever step I took towards our door made me feel like I was leaving pieces of me behind. The cap on my head had bored its way through. Rest was going to be my only resort but the pain only dissipated after many hours of resting. I met a new beast from the airport, one that curtailed my getting into vehicles for quite a while.

I sacrificed health to attend my niece's wedding and like the airport, the return trip was an ordeal, I couldn't risk another. The good part about pain, if you can see good in bad, is that it is a warning of something More Stark looming. The more pain the More Severe the threat and we ought to listen to our body's screams. As important as it may be to be there for a wedding, there is greater importance in being here for the marriage. It was My Sacrifice, misguided as it was, because, not listening to the screams from my body could have meant hushing its whispers. I was opening the doors to greater demise. The slightest rupture in nerves due to continuous harsh stimulation, can lead to permanent damage. Seeing the wedding ceremony might be blissful but seeing the fruit of their union, the children born of the couple, would be much more meaningful. My grandniece came soon after their marriage and will be six years this year. I think there is a blessing to meet a new generation and for them to meet us. There is much that can pass between generations. She saw me regularly from nursing days, Me Sitting the same place each time and was shock to see Me Standing for the first time, when she was four. I hope I can surprise here in other good ways later. It is because of this continuation of life as new generations are born, that we owe it to each other to pay closer attention to our health. To listen to those screams inside us, slay our dragons and hush our demons. Surely the dogma, "If thy foot offends you, cut it off" doesn't elicit a similar response, should the head behave the same.

The car rides made my head feel like it was my biggest burden. All other troubles paled at the time and I felt to be rid of it. But, desires born from agony are pleads for mercy like shouts of anguish, unmeasured and untrue. In rational times we recognize what these uncontrolled words imply but when pain and anguish overwhelm us, rationality and reasoning die.

If we can overcome these harsh times, remembering the adage "This too will pass" then we can thrust our swords into our dragons and live tomorrow to wield them again.

I'll stand, thank you!

When he diagnosed a horrid and possibly brief future, my doctor also suggested treatment was going to be a financial strain and recommended I seek help through Public Healthcare. He cautioned me that although I might not pay in money, I would pay in the time waiting. His care and appointment scheduling were unmatched and it was going to be a Major Sacrifice to be without them but he was right, the medical bills climbed too high. The maintenance for medication alone was contributing BDS$3,000 monthly. It was a hill too steep to climb on my existing salary. When I discovered shortly afterwards the company no longer needed My Skills, medication was an impossible expense. I had no choice but to downscale to public care.

The description I had from my private doctor didn't quite prepare me for what was ahead. Yes, my first hour waiting was already 45 minutes longer than I ever waited at my doctor. By the time three hours had passed, I was weak with exhaustion, hungry and scared a seizure was looming. Then I heard my name called and felt at least 10 pairs of eyes on me, from a room of about 15 people, reduced from the 50 that were waiting 2 hours before.

hen I started taking the medication, dosages were to be 48 hours apart and the regiment of alternate days at 9:00 a.m. began. My Seizures where not triggered by any known means and I traced it only to my body being spent. The dilemma of clashing clinic appointments with the administration of medication times, together with my uncertain onset of seizures, escalated beyond me. I tried to discuss special arrangements with the attendant nurses, that they might receive me after 9:30 and allow me timely admission to the doctor. They tried and for the next four visits I waited 1 hour the most, but the doctors kept their own tardy schedules and soon I was back to 3 and more hours wait. I would arrive to clinic for 9:30 and never leave until 1:00 p.m. the earliest. Patients tended to arrive as early as 8:00 a.m. so as to assure their seating. I never could imagine how the elderly and sick were expected to wait these hours pass lunch time with signs saying "No Eating" posted on the walls. How were the diabetics fearing and what about people who had to eat before their midday medication? I heard all kinds of stories in those clinic chairs with unexpected wisdom. I took away stories but could never carry names or faces long enough to describe the storytellers. Fortunately for me, not everyone has anomic aphasia or suffers any degree of prosopagnosia. Recognizing me, some caring elderly people would offer their seats minutes after I arrived and rotated between them to prevent me from being on my feet too long. They were perceptive, More So it seemed than the nurses who should have been able to read my condition slipping away as I waited. If standing for over fifteen minutes, I could feel a slicing pain separating my lower back and losing my ability to stand. My legs would get like rubber bands and offer no support. I tried to not grimace and I looked away so as not to have begging eyes.

I am and will be eternally grateful to those strangers who stood up that I May Sit, who despite their own personal demons, got to their feet that I might get off Mine Still voluntarily. Walks on mornings got Me Stronger and my legs grew more accustomed to being in a vertical position. Soon, I was able to stand for longer periods and my trips to clinic were not as burdensome. When I arrived to clinic one morning, an elderly lady who recognized me from a previous visit offered me her seat. For the first time, I was able to say with a generous smile of gratification, I'll stand, thank you!

I still visit clinic on their time schedule and fortunately I find seating in other rooms when our room is overcrowded. The wait is still very long but as I sit, I recall the many other times when to be awake was to remember seizures and the fear of being alone was imagining something tragic about to happen. Now, I can sit fearless of time forcing dark clouds and just observe the blessing of seeing faces, previously blank from failed vision. The time waiting in clinic is used for introspection and supposition. I also talk gently to patients and listen attentively. The clinic experience, with all its ordeal, no longer presents a problem. I go with the expectation that I will have to wait for hours and prepare new comers for the same.

My Somewhat recluse life does not afford regular meetings with anyone other than caregivers. Patients come in all ages, sizes and sexes and for the time I have been going to clinic, I met new friends and saw some old ones. I had some short reunions with people long lost in my past, short meetings that revealed more of their lives than the many years I had known them. The reality of impending demise brings out an open honesty in people. At dust, the sunset can be beautiful and these patients approaching their dust can shine wonderfully. Sometimes the best sunsets are only visible beyond thicket of bushes and trees. Once we get past the obstructing veneer, the protective shields people wore for many years and lowered as the dust of their lives approaches, we get to see yet another of our many blessings, the hearts of people.

We learn so much when we wait patiently, observing the realities around us and recognizing we are but a miniscule part of a whole. Like the microbes of a being, we have a role to play. Our contribution when measured against the infinite roles of others, seems insignificant but it bears up the whole. A single drop of ocean that traveled from the North to the South Pole and still remained a single drop, hidden in the vastness of the whole but contributing in its singular role. I don't know what consequences my brief conversation with fellow patients has on them but I know their brief act of kindness, smile or simple gesture hello, melts away the ordeal of clinic.

The wait of three hours for three minutes with doctors is no longer a burdensome

abuse of time.

Before I go

When you got here, to this place, to read this page, I hope you were not like me. I

took My Sight for granted, never imagined the possibility of not being able to see.

I lived guilty of misgivings and expectant that some things will always be the same.

The simple things that came easily like smiling, walking, running, talking, breathing,

writing and seeing, the whole list of them, I took them all for granted. I lived life

to the fullest. Never to the fullest as defined by the activities of thrill seekers

and spaced out bingers. No, I felt complete with happiness of a different kind and

got my highs day and night, but not highs that left Me So depleted, like a junky I

craved the next. I moved between highs with little down time, after two hours

sleep, I was ready to go again.

Work absorbed me fully and took away all other life. I was happy to do it, showed

up early on mornings and left late at night. It's funny how I got so caught in

misguided loyalties, I lost sight of salient priorities. Work became my mistress and

soon she was My Spouse. She bore me thousands of children, my clients, and my

devotion to them was unrelenting. I lived to serve them and smiled each time I did.

It was never about the money, they never paid me enough, nor was it power, My Superiors kept the reins tight. Like any loyal parent, I was happy and satisfied to watch my children grow in their successes. In my twenty years of management, I recall only two children who scoffed my way, and like a good shepherd whose lamb wonders off from his care, it pained me when I couldn't lead them back to gratification.

The unusual commitment to my profession, categorized me as a workaholic but that is far from true. I have always been overly committed, whether it was school or work. I never missed a day of school from Combermere, just like I never took days off from work. My health was never in question and I was there to answer every roll call. Perhaps that was wrong, I know now my going out could have inflicted others.

At my final workplace we kept regular Friday meetings, fashioned from an imported custom called "Beer Talks." I spoke against beers and we decided to keep clearer heads with nonalcoholic drinks. I convinced my colleagues our talks should be "Bare

Talks" where staff could come freely and bare their true feelings about the week's happenings without fear of victimization.

I was having a very high fever over the weekend after clearing out one of our warehouses, the Friday. I might have over exposed myself to the mounds of bat droppings and years of piling dust, or so I self-diagnosed. A scheduled trip for two of my fellow managers would take them away at a critical time but I agreed to do the appraisals with a supervisor's assistance. My Stupid misguided loyalty prevented me from more rational judgment and caused me to show up to work, despite a burning fever. I sat through three days of appraisal meetings with the staff and was able to give my colleagues complete assessments when they returned. Three weeks later I was in an ophthalmologist's office and three weeks following that, a neurologist was examining me for a condition my negligence and misdirected priorities, may have caused.

The diagnosis of Multiple Sclerosis follows a garrison of tests but none of them can confirm why a person is afflicted. Experts have narrowed possible causes to three general reasons.

My doctor eliminated hereditary since there is no historical evidence I would have any genetic predisposition to the kinds of environmental agents that might trigger autoimmune responses. I have no family prior with MS.

A second contributor for MS seems to be geographical location with the general consensus being that MS in more prevalent in countries with temperate climates. Epidemiological evidence support the theory that the further from the equator, the more common the disease. There is a higher prevalence in Scandinavian countries and northern Europe than in Latin American. Race is also associated with geographical proximity and generally, Whites in the US are more prone than Blacks. There was no reason why my MS should be geographically associated either.

The doctor was never and still has never been able to associate my MS. The final cause is viral and no one to date has verified the theory that some viruses bring on MS. I do not discount the complex virus's ability and favor this clinical postulation, especially since on the eve of being diagnosed with this lifelong illness, I had a terrifically high fever from a head cold and was also exposed to the dirt and grime which accumulated over a decade, in that filthy warehouse. My Studies from school, together with specific bits of information, lead me to my own conclusion. I am far from being medically qualified to formulate a viable thesis but by way of qualification, I listen closely to whispered Messages Spoken spiritually, and I follow their guidance since similar messages have proven in my favor. A virus can lay dormant for many years in a state similar to the chrysalis of butterflies, only it doesn't have to nourish. The virus stays dormant until favorable conditions are met, where it invades its host and takes over cellular encoding, making healthy body cells bend to its will.

I believe my extremely high fever made the membranes in my brain cells more permeable to viral activity and they migrated into My Spinal cord where they launch attacks against my nerves. This theory is supported by some medical practitioners and is not as bogus as one would imagine, coming from its unschooled source.

There is no real proof what caused me to get MS but finding out has not been My

Struggle. I will help the cause to ascertain why people get MS and to prevent

people being afflicted with this disease but a greater cause and more urgent need

is how we deal with it. I choose to treat my MS as Mock Sport, where, My Senses

are given untrue and often unrealistic advice to react to changes in the environs

that are false. My dedication and loyalty is no longer misdirected but rather, is

focused on living from My Soul. My legs don't take me about freely, but I strive to

give legs to My Spirit and quieten the demon that invaded my body.

Before I go, I want My Spirit to pour out its truths and to share My Story.

Do you say posthumously fluently?

I shudder at the thought of what Hollywood perpetuates happens to us at death. The glamourized, return visits of loved ones to finalized unfinished business, like in Ghost Whisper, or the light leading to deceased loved ones, waiting, welcoming with opened arms. I enjoy with tears their fictitious accounts of possibility even though I recognize the impossible premise. Like everyone I know, a visit from one who was "Gone too soon" though creepy, would be useful closure. To know what they truly felt in that final time, when lies have taken vacation and promises are said with real earnest. The final time when we get to see the true person and have a real heart to heart. I too crave these unguarded moments and shed tears when I see them played out in fantasy.

I said I was a TV enthusiast, I know lots would say a TV tick. I soaked up quite a few series over the years. Never had a reading hobby, which was bad, My Schooling suffered from this lack of reading skill. I still don't read much, which is weird coming from someone who writes these long essays, hoping to share them, and hoping you read them in full. Those getting this far in this one must have read some of the previous ones already since you obvious are not as averse as I am, to long scrolling paragraphs. I see words sometimes and run. One lady told Me She started to read and when she clicked on "see more," though she was interested in what would follow, she was intimidated by the many long paragraphs ahead and close it, disappointed in not getting to reach the conclusion, left with unanswered questions. The answers were right there within view but the climb was too steep.

Charles Ingalls from the "Little House on the Prairie" was the ideal man in the Hollywood role and later I found out, Michael Landon who played the part was an incredible person too. In Season 1, Episode 6, 1974: If I Should Wake Before I Die, certain that only her funeral would bring her distant children and their children to Walnut Grove, Amy desperate to celebrate her eightieth birthday reacquainting with her family, convinces Doc Baker and Charles to fake her death and plan her funeral. This episode had a vital message then but its reality was only revealed to me now my glory days are behind. I want to be able to snatch Hollywood's fantasies and make them real, to speak openly and from the heart to those who care to listen and share in earnest, true feelings. I want to say I love you and have it understood and believed. Perhaps Hollywood is right and there will be a brief moment to have these sincere chats but why must it be closure and goodbye? Why can't we speak with each other now, unguarded, fearless of being trampled on, used or abused? If a person's attitude is one you love and admire, why can't it be shared, just as we share the negative things we see in each other?

Recently, I have been getting very moving comments from my Facebook friends, many in private inbox but often bold and public. These FB friends have shown their preparedness to give me that Hollywood fantasy of openness. The truths of their hearts and I know it doesn't come easily, exposing your depth publicly, so when you do, know how much it is admired. I lived to enjoy my TV fantasies without waiting until that final passage. I see the outstretched arms welcoming these long rants and learn of you sharing them with others you believe may be inspired.

MS took My Senses and has done with them as it wishes but My Soul, My Spirit, My Strength nourished by My Saviour have brought me this far, and have given me this opportunity to see the unforced good nature of Many Strangers and My friendS.

I experience NOW the accolades and gestures of kindness with your gracious comments, and can say with sincerity and truthfulness, they are fully appreciated. I don't know what will be said posthumously and could never answer them, but I love you NOW!

Fighting demons

My Sister deserted her home next door to take up residency with me. Alana wanted to be even closer should I need immediate help. She guarded my room as I slept amidst protective pillows she had placed around me, like a baby. There was the chance of seizures in My Sleep and she sought to cushion me from uncontrolled, self-inflicted damage. We were in the living room one evening when she asked me to pass her the remote. I have heard of males' reluctance to give up the controls but I had no reservation to giving her. Her exceptional taste in movies and unselfish desire to share, always landed us on something we had mutual taste in and could enjoy.

When I clasped my hand to take it up, I thought I had grabbed a five pound weight. The remote was inexplicably heavy and we laughed at my flawed judgment. The next morning I tried to turn in bed but got no assistance from my right arm. It chose to stay limped and asleep. I fought the rest of my body to an upright position and watched as the right arm fell to My Side.

Accustomed to trips to the doctor, there was no mad rush. Daddy brought my breakfast tray as had been his custom for weeks. I knew I wasn't going to have the aid of my right arm and prepared to use the left. I smiled at its clumsiness. It couldn't find the way to my lips with a spoonful of cereal without spilling half. The mug of hot honey was easier to manage and my dad sat across the room watching me finish. Almost done, with only a banana left, tears flooded my eyes. I was pondering on how to peel the banana and for the first time, completely realized the importance of a functional right arm. I tried to laugh with what little bravery was left but the thought of not having the right arm to use on many other tasks only brought streaming tears.

I got readmitted and more tests were scheduled. I was to get MRIs of the brain and neck, to pinpoint what my doctor suspected. A very close friend went with me and was in the room, sitting to the right of the huge chamber. The technician had already checked we had no metal objects and briefed us of the machine's operation. I was to lie still, after being injected with a dye when she determined through tests, I had no fish allergies. It was amazing how the injection streamed through the body in such a short space of time. There in the chamber, the repeated clicking, clanging sounds overwhelmed the background music played to sooth and took control of my helpless hand, which developed its own pulsing. I couldn't control the shaking and my friend moved over to My Side and held my arm steady. I felt the comfort of her presence. Her gentle, consoling touch lulled me to sleep despite the disturbing noise.

The MRIs confirmed what my doctor had suspected and he gave me the news that evening. A blood clot was discovered in the base of my brain. The clot was in a vessel which drains the brain and was not very life threatening, nor of the More Serious kind. Once dislodge, they expected return use of my arm and better mobility. It was comforting news but the coming days had shown no real change. The therapist beat my arm to beckon it move but the only response was in feeling her slaps. Every morning she came, she offered hope and went about her routine with the zealousness that each new day was the day for change. Each day she was the same, even when she saw no response, still ripe with expectation and a warm, concerned demeanor. Every evening I saw the faces of my family with hopes dwindling and tears in my father's eyes.

During the day, in my alone time, I looked at the arm that had been beaten hours before and showed no retaliation. I thought of all My Stubborn ways, all the times I refused to fall in line with tradition and wanted to do things my way. I remembered My Sweetheart at school who when asked by a teacher to spell stubborn, how she bloated out "A D R I A N!" I could recall sharing the single bedroom with my parents and two older siblings and Me Stubbornly wanting to say my prayers before climbing into bed, not knowing the words, but insisting I could. I recalled memories of stubborn me, reasons plausible, but stubborn none the less. The many times I boastfully told people I was proudly stubborn in my ways because I truly believe what I did to be right. Now, my arm was being a stubborn appendage of me and I was getting a dose of what it feels like, not knowing why the refusal to conform.

The therapist thought she saw a flicker one morning and was even more determined. The slaps were harder and more vigorous, then I saw it too. The little finger hinted an involuntary motion and moved just enough to show a single tremor. This grown man cried again, from joy this time and thanked the therapist with profuse gratitude.

I smiled all day and kept the secret from my family, to release it on their visit. My mom and sister had grown used to massaging my arm and I had even guided them on how to continue the therapy I had been taught. That evening when my mom was going through the routine and conversation was flowing in the room, she stopped and they hushed when I announced I had something to show them.

My palm was faced down at the side of the bed and I asked them to watch. The motion was so small you needed to look closely but it was not so small that expectant eyes, hanging on desperate hopes, couldn't perceive. The room was like the ball had been dropped on Times Square. Screams of joys burst the solemn corridors of the private ward and brought nurses running. They shared the joy too but offered a polite hush, "You must keep it down." The elation of progress was like the dawn of a new day. My family's faces were radiant and my dad's tears subsided, displaced with a smile of contentment. It wasn't long afterwards that the arm responded completely. New MRIs showed a reduction in the clot.

I went home and only then did I realize, vibrations brought excruciating pain which made my head feel like it was locked in a vice and the tightening wheels were turning. The motor of the car brought it on. The fans in the house, the electric can opener, kitchen appliances, any motor contributed to my pain. Living around me was like walking on eggshells but my family was patient and accommodating. They abandoned many of their habits that I Might Survive my ordeal with minimum annoyance. I was worse than the miserable old lady we fretted as kids, who lived across the road and never wanted us to shout in play. I couldn't believe the number of things we used that had disturbing motors. For months I didn't cut my hair because of the motor, and my right arm was not dexterous enough for a pair of scissors. It took almost a year of use before I was finally able to write legibly again, longer to sign.

A blood clot can be miniscule but its effect on the body enormous. These little dams of destruction pose great risk of life to us all and it is hard to predict clots. Our lifestyles do not prohibit their danger and if prone to clots, doctors may put you on the rat poison "Warfin" and keep you on regular INR (International Normalized Ratio) tests to monitor that proper ratio of blood cells and platelets is maintained. But our diets have their own blood thinners and close scrutiny of what we eat can naturally balance the blood's INR. Due largely to the unpredictability of my clots, activity is carefully watched, no pricks or slits, no scratches or slashes. I'm like a house of cards, maintained with delicacy. Flossing can introduce dangerous bleeding and consequently, I am generally refused by dentists.

Today, I am free of the devastating clot on my brain and of discomfort in my head from motors. We fought that demon together, my family and I, and together, one year later, we fought another perilous clot in my lungs, the dreaded pulmonary embolism. My high risk for these potentially fatal clots has determined the bland diet I adhered to these last 10 years. I hear the frustrated patients in clinic who stray from their diets for temporary sweet and learn of their troubles of fluctuating, poor health. I see how desperate people can be to restore their eating pleasure and how indifferent they treat the inability to balance their INR. People who defy medical advice to be pleasured for just a moment. My Stubbornness kicks in again and although my mom, my cook, would love to change menu for the sake of variety, I am happy to stay fixed on bland.

A moment's pleasure at the expense of better health is never a good trade off.

Tossing and shaking violently

When I regained balance, sufficient to walk freely, I continued the regiment of exercises the therapist had taken me through, confident they worked. During the day I took Measured Steps through the house, using the walls only when necessary to steady me and of course avert any falls. I had tried going outside in the road before but it only served to amuse my neighbor. When I opened the gate to head left, I was prepared to go the 50 yards to the end of our gap, turn and return to our gate, thus completing an approximate 100 yards. I figured if I could do that, I would have a better count of my progress with repeated and additional cycles. This wasn't to be. As soon as I closed the gate behind me, I completed three steps and could go no further. I wish I could fully describe what the sensation is like, when your mind can no longer command your legs to move, even when your legs feel energized to walk. The gradual filling up of phantom sand in my legs, weighing them down so heavily, lifting was too strenuous. I turned and dragged my legs back to my gate and my neighbor watched every night when I tried at around the same time, each time managing to add one step.

During the day I walked the length of the house and counted My Steps until my legs were too heavy to carry me. My Sister got me a pedometer that later did the counting for me and before long, I was doing so Many Steps in the house, I tackled the road again, this time on early mornings. I didn't go until my legs were too heavy, I used the pedometer and my alarm clock to measure both distance and time. I felt accomplished when I was able to walk freely in the road, with steps climbing from 500 to 1000s, from 30 minutes to 2 hours of continuous walk. I felt so revved and boastful, everyone who sat long enough would learn of my accomplishments. Soon, my walks were the talk from neighbors' lips. I started around 4:00 a.m. and finished at 6:00 a.m. A stringent Medication Schedule dictated breakfast time and therefore my cut off. Some days I felt I could go more. Those days I took the walk to the beach. I still needed to stay away from the direct rays of the sun, which felt like they were baking My Skin, even when exposed for only seconds to early Morning Sunlight. The hotter I got the less I could see. Everything would become like shadows, somewhat like when we stared into the sun, for fun, as kids.

I used to recall the times and date quickly, but the morning I felt like all was going backwards, when My Steps were staggered and shaky again, seems to elude me now. The sensation I felt, forced me to go back inside. I had become so shaken, I cancelled my beach date to rest instead.

But rest didn't come easily. I didn't want this set back, not after I had been doing so well. My gradual progress had made Me So efficient, I could stand in the doctors' offices when there were no chairs, for 30 minutes before crisis point, or stand while waiting to be collected. There was a sense of independence when I was no longer compelled to accept the offer of a seat, from blatantly older people who themselves were ill. They would detect my discomfort and though bent with age, would painfully get up and insist I sit. It had been Months Since my face and body could betray my desire for independence and that was triumphant. Victory was nearing, "Land ahoy, skipper!"

I knew the nature of the beast I faced. I knew Relapsing-Remitting Multiple Sclerosis (RRMS) is the most common of the four types of MS, initially diagnosed in approximately 85 percent of MS patients. I read you should expect the disease course to take defined attacks of worsening magnitude followed by partial or complete recovery periods. I also knew that relapses generally lead to dwindling recovery, either none at all or the returned ability was more deficient. I had seen this already with My Sight. My vision never returned to the 20/16 it was, in fact, it was more like 200/35, about 70 percent recovered. I may have these figures all wrong but suffice it to say, as happy as I was to finally make out faces again and see the color of flowers in the gardens, I was no longer near my previous ability to read a computer monitor from across the room. I can't see the video or pictures in most phones. Given all this, I should have been better emotionally prepared for relapses.

The ground in the gap was vibrating beneath my feet and my unsteadiness was like walking a rocking boat. The feeling was familiar and disturbing. My progress seemed to have relapsed but that point didn't get home as clearly to me as later in the morning while in bed. I seldom go back to bed for rest and when I do, my family are immediately aware something is wrong. My mom was in the yard when I felt like my body was having convulsions. I remained conscious and when I looked down at my legs, I saw the bed moving. Straight off I thought it was a worsening of my relapsing episodes. I experienced spinning rooms before, this was a crude variation. It was hard to climb from the moving bed but I needed to get to my parents since I hadn't yet relearned how to project my voice. The passageways I walked in my home so often were hard to maneuver. I slid my hand along the wall for support and could feel everything vibrating beneath my touch. The vibrations seemed to cause the wall hangings to dance. This was appearing to be my worse episode ever. When I finally got to my dad in his room, he stared franticly at me. His fear had his hair standing. He grabbed onto the bed and shouted in a wavering, scared voice, "You feel that?" Almost with his question, it stopped and a reassuring smile burst into a laugh. He was feeling the vibration too. I wasn't getting a bad episode. We heard mommy using the washing machine and thought the impractical, that the spin cycle was shaking the house badly. A news bulletin corrected us. It announced Barbados had experienced earth tremors from a quake off the island.

The news never explained the vibrations I experienced hours before the tremors that had Me So shaken, I staggered returning home and cancelled the beach. I believe My Senses are more acute and I can easily suffer from slight variations in the ambience, like off balancing with a gentle breeze. Animals through their augmented sensors, can detect slight seismographic changes and get to safe ground before the actual earth tremors. Perhaps my legs sensed these vibration that morning early.

It seems all the tossing and violent shaking did something to me because, I wasn't able to walk steadily for years afterwards. In fact, I still haven't gotten back to the progress I had made. It was a very gradual process before. One single step added each day, led to thousands of steps eventually. I had used this gradual process of incrementing to achieve many other feats and move some mountains, a bucket at a time. We can achieve most our goals with steady application of increasing growth. Pay yourself a single dollar for every movie you watch, every song you listen to and every time you wish people had shown more kindness or thoughtfulness. See the growth you make over a year.

I shall increment additional steps again daily if it would mean reaching that level of independence, when I could say, "No thank you!" to the offer of a seat. And if one small gesture daily brings a smile, then daily I shall build smiles and pray each smile warms the heart of the person smiling and that those looking on, would catch its warmth and pass it on too.

I will sow the little seeds of treasured MomentS and reap the abundance of pleasurable MemorieS.

50

Letting Go

I had a seizure in the bath early morning before My Shower. I felt something

strange about to happen and when my right arm started to float uncontrollably

from My Side, I was convinced something was already happening. I tried to lower it

with the left but couldn't. My Shout to my parents was more of fear than for help.

Daddy was in the kitchen and Mummy Still in bed but they both heard and came

running to see my then unconscious, naked body in seizures on the floor. They tried

to tell me what they saw but neither could get composure enough to utter

coherency. I could hear their fear but couldn't imagine what they must have gone

through, watching their seemingly invincible son in helpless, involuntary contortions.

They did say I was heavy to carry. When I came through I was on their bed and we

talked about going back to the doctor.

It seemed like everything was happening so speedily after my first visit; like my

body was surrendering without a fight and took no consultation with me. I lost

control and agreed I should return. I had started taking medications prescribed

and was having side effects which became obvious with the rash and sores down my arms. On my visit, the doctor changed the Medication Suspected and warned me against its use or other near derivatives. He wanted to keep me for further observation and tests, so I went to the reception area to be admitted.

Mommy Saw me in while daddy parked the car but as she was going out to him, I caught her at the door with my outcry, "It's happening again!" I know the folk in the lobby were shocked at my outburst. They saw no apparent physical crisis, but I felt my right arm starting to float. The doctor's advice still minutes fresh was loud in my head. "Next time he has a seizure don't move him, turn him to his right side and support his head." I lowered myself and assumed the position before losing consciousness, just in time to hear the archaic screams behind the front counter, "Put something in his mouth!" Thankfully my mother was in with the doctor and knew these front desk hospital staff were uninformed and their frantic suggestion was not procedural. You can't swallow your tongue, worst case scenario you may bite it but you do that even when conscious. It was the least of concerns. Mommy cradled my head in her lap as the 30 seconds passed. It was a little longer than previous and I didn't get fully conscious until they had taken me to a room and hooked me up to many monitors.

In an unconscious state I heard someone praying over me. We were alone and his words, though hazy, seemed very sincere. I could not get an image, my eyes were still close but the male voice was etched in me. When I opened my eyes, still a bit disoriented, my mother was sitting by my bedside and her words were soft in whispers and solemnly sweet. It doesn't matter that I can't remember what she was saying, it matters that she was there, helping me understand this new world I opened my eyes to, like at my birth. All around me was strange and might have been frightening had she not been there, either time. She assured me there were no bugs crawling on my face and helped me to water which soothed my parchedness. After the quenching, I became aware of My Surroundings. It was like rain from a cloud, emotions burst and overwhelmed me, but there were no tears. I struggled to be brave, especially before my mom who had seemed so defeated earlier that morning when she saw the first seizure. Now, a second and worse one, followed by the machines and hospitalization. But My Struggle ended when the etched male's voice emerged in my consciousness and a great reassurance came over me.

I know it was harder for others looking on since they could not hear My Soul. Inside, it sang and trumpeted defeat. It assured me the time had not yet come and many days ahead were awaiting me. There were going to be trying times, worse than had been, but My Spirit had already grown strong and I natured it more in the quiet of my room. There on the hospital bed, I was getting stronger physically and in days, I was able to walk unaided, but growing at a more exponential curve, My Spirit was already soaring.

To proceed in this new life I woke to, I needed to let go the memories of the other life. The ones that could bind chains about you and prevent you from going beyond the unnecessary constructs of doctors and caregivers. Our bodies write the pages of medical journals not doctors, they just record scripts for others to read. We provide the material to study and who knows which of our bodies will write the treatments and cures for baffling ailments. Letting go was easy. I wanted to let my new life be a guide and not a consequence. I wanted for people to see me beyond My Shell and realize that I awoke after that seizure to the reality that my problems at work no longer mattered. The crises which plagued my thoughts before I dropped to the floor in that reception lounge, disappeared when I opened my eyes to a new acceptance of what I was limited to do physically. My Spirit was limitless.

Recently, your comments assured me My Sedate life, here at home can still be meaningful. It is safe to release the chains that bind you to limitations of the past and soar. There is no time better than now.

Letting go of the past is made easier when we reach out and grasp the truth of our reality and step bravely into the future.

Tunnel Vision

The symptoms I was experiencing warranted a visit to the specialist who asked

questions I might have needed Tony and Doug to help me with.

If you are a TV dinosaur then you might remember the 10 years old government

secret project "Tic toc" that was threatened with cancellation after what

appeared to be billions of squandered funds. The project was to build and

experimental time machine called the "Time Tunnel." They had not perfected its

operations yet but the visiting Senator in charge of funding, insisted to see it in

action. While Doug was convincing him they were not ready, Tony launched himself

through the time machine. Doug learned of his colleague's rambunctiousness, and

went immediately to bring him back, but the two doctors were transferred into

different times and places. This Sci-Fi series misjudged the progression of man's

scientific aptitude since it was based in 1968, just one year ahead of its filming

and there was no likelihood of time travel in that millennium or this. At least Star

Trek gave us a bit more time to achieve the technologies it featured. Although we still have not reached the "Teleports" to cry "Beam me up Scotty," cordless communication, video phones, a global information centre (Internet), and many other gadgets and ideas from the show have been realized.

In the Time Tunnel, the doctors were lost but could be seen in a video impression cast on the tunnel. It was also possible for the home team to communicate with Doug and Tony or send them tangible help. In their travels, the doctors visited the sinking Titanic, D Day Pearl Harbor, the eruption of Krakatoa, battle at the Alamo and many other historical thresholds during separate episodes.

When the doctor asked if I had been struck on my head, I suspect he was trying to attribute the double vision, I could have used a visual implement into my past, a Time Tunnel perhaps. At that time it was hard to remember recent knocks to my head. I could recall siting under the window of Mr. Jones's class at Wesley Hall Primary School, watching "Hardball" cricket and catching a well-played six on the top of my head." When I was younger, while watching the "Big boys" pelting at some hog plums, the big yellow ones that grow high in a tree, I was standing too close. The pull back of "Tiptoe's" action was abruptly stopped by the top of my head and the big rock opened my cranium, which bled profusely. The boys rushed me to my grandmother, mum and she used her all curing "Cou-cou" on it. These all happened before I was 10 years old so they could hardly be responsible for My Symptoms 30 years later. I tried to but could not remember recent blows to my head, so the doctor took new directions for causation.

My ophthalmologist hinted possibilities and proposed the likelihood of Myasthenia Gravis, when scheduling an appointment for me. Her speculations prompted me to read up as much material as I could to become acquainted with this unwelcomed, lifelong companion. MG is akin to MS, both being autoimmune diseases but this cousin may best be described as the body fighting against its own muscular tissue and not like its kin MS where the fight is taken to the nerves. You can see how they would have similar Motor Symptoms, and why at a glance, they can be easily mistaken even by trained eyes. The Neurologist, having a closer intimacy with the nerves was quick to eliminate MG and when he said people tended not to contract its cousin MS in their 40's, I inwardly smiled. I thought these lifelong ailments were not diseases ravaging my body and more calmly I prepared for a treatable diagnosis and to be rid of these Menacing Symptoms.

In my unguarded misdirection, I didn't recall the instances in my teenage life that may have been telling signs. I laughed at my alopecia areata because that single bald spot, no bigger than a dollar coin, was supposed to have been caused by my girlfriend who claimed knowledge of witch craft. Also, during those more gullible years at sixteen, I was having peripheral sight problems during a school day. I told the hockey coach I wasn't going to be able to play in the game that evening and a school mate asked me to describe what I was experiencing. I told him it was like looking through a pipe, I was only seeing what was focally in front of me. I actually described it as tunnel vision. "Cornguts" couldn't fully understand but suggested it was probably hunger and I should have a heavy lunch with rest during the lunch break. It was considerate of Bostic and I took his advice.

This tunnel vision went away by late evening, after the game. It returned once more, months afterwards but never again. On reflection, and having read some of the early signs for related diseases, perhaps MS was making and early call on me. Few if anyone, understood the disease before the mid 80's, so I couldn't have been diagnosed back then. In fact, here is an unwitting play on words. Prior to Pryor, I mean the actor Richard Pryor's diagnosis of MS, I never even heard of Multiple Sclerosis or its family of illnesses, like Lupus and MG.

Tony and Doug had been lost is the Time Tunnel as their home team of great technical minds bounced them through changing continuums. The tunnel vision I experienced then would have only been a sign to a select, present neurologists, so I didn't miss early prevention. Any changing signs, how ever nogligible they may appear today, are likely signals you ought to pay closer attention to. Don't ignore your body if it cries out. Hunger is the cry of a body already in crisis, we should avoid getting hungry by eating at conditioned times. Don't wait until something screams inside of you to act or do what you know you ought to have done. Pay very close attention to your body and do not wait until it cries. Believe it or not, thirst is a scream from the body that it is dehydrating. Drink regularly, don't wait until you are thirsty. A dehydrated body can go into shock and have permanent damage to vital organs. They still can't say definitively what brought on my MS but like many other ailments, an imbalance of the internal environ can lead to over acidity in the tissues, resulting in cellular activity going chaotic. Healthy cells can attack each other or nearby cells. Just low cellular water levels can result in the diffusion of passersby that might otherwise have just passed by. They gain admission into critical cells and later refuse to get out. It's all getting too complicated but bear in mind, these are simple cells conditioned to perform a set role. By just allowing ourselves to become dehydrated, inebriated, or any of a litany of "ateds" we could experience a complete change in our quality of health. Tunnel vision isn't a bad thing if we heed the good word from the Proverbs, chapter 4:25 "Let thine eyes look right on, and let thine eyelids look straight before thee." Stay focus and don't be distracted by what we see left or right. Look straight ahead through your tunnel and walk, providing of course you are focused on the positive and righteous. I didn't know if my episode was a telltale sign then and no medical knowledge at that time would have. What it should have taught me then is that I needed to focus, stay focus and walk a straight path. Perhaps it would have saved me from all those dead ends and wrong turns I made later. My tunnel vision may be clinically interpreted by the medical fraternity now as telltale signs of MS and with newly armed medical wisdom, be conclusive. Looking back at it, metaphorically for me it was a signal of impending wisdom and attitude, ignored through boyish ignorance.

In hindsight, I'm seeing it now as a learning moment that given the Time Tunnel, I would have made better use of it.

My Spinal tap

I left the doctor's office trying to learn to pronounce My Suspected condition and understand what and why I should be diagnosed with this Acute disseminated encephalomyelitis (ADE). My ophthalmologist had referred me to a Neurologist when she realized the double vision in my right eye was likely nerve damage. She indicated my loss of vision could not be corrected with glasses and scheduled an urgent appointment on my behalf.

The specialist would see me within 3 weeks the soonest so in the interim, I drove knowing I couldn't depend on a right glance, close my right eye to see on that side. The contortions of my neck though awkward, gave Me Such a release to see accurately what the traffic was really like and made me feel Much Safer making my go decisions from junctions.

I worked during the 3 weeks and continued my dancing appointment on Sundays. On appointment day, a Thursday, the doctor took what seemed a casual look but to his trained eye and astute qualifications, detailed enough to confirm more invasive checks required. He scheduled me for the coming Tuesday, timing I thought was incredibly soon given the difficulty with getting to see him in the first place. But, time dragged its slowest and conditions escalated with unwarranted acceleration. The sock like numbness had climbed from my ankles to above my knees and my legs took on their own direction, refusing to make coordinated placement to move me forward. I fought to get alternating left right rhythms and to stay on a straight course. My face felt like I had cobweb and brushing and washing it never helped. I didn't go to dancing that Sunday and the arrangement made earlier to take my mom to watch a performance at the People's Cathedral was going to be cancelled, except, one of her friends volunteered to take us both. That night, stepping out of the car was like jumping hurdles with no training while wearing stilts. The ladies helped me into the church when we realized walking the grass pavement and the downward sloping path were equally foreign and challenging for me. I felt like a baby now discovering its legs but must have looked like an intoxicated bibber.

By the time I got into the doctor's office that Tuesday, I was like he noticed in his casual glance, "Adrian, you are a completely different case today." Facial dysphagia had drooped the left side of my face and I could neither make a grin or a smile.

Shucks, I always had trouble "steupsing" after having the habit knocked out of me

by the Math teacher in second form, but now, my lips couldn't form the pouting

required and my tongue had become too lazy to move comfortably on command. At

the end of his rigorous tests he admitted me to private hospital and set up further

testing. It was an afternoon visit when he told me of the need for a lumbar tap. He

was quiet and I was speechless with a greater fear than had been looming since the

uncertainty of My Sickness. In every figment of my imagination and deep in my

core, the knowledge of this dreaded intrusion by the huge needle into the spine

was the pain that surpassed all others. The doctor didn't warn me of any of the

potential dangers and was seemly nonchalant about my impending pain. He said he

would return to do the test that evening which gave me about 4 hours. Perhaps it

was good I had so little time to ponder my trepidation. Before I could swelter in

fear he was back. The nurse was not helpful and actually was prepping me

unsuitably for the doctor. He came in and corrected her and assured me it was not

going to take long. I told him, given the associated pain, I know I couldn't bear it

any longer than moments. He smiled and again nonchalantly, said it's only a prick.

I had seen the tests done on television and it was always the same, turn on a side and be as steady as possible amidst excruciating pain. Mentally prepared, I got on My Side when the doctor came and backed him. I didn't even want to see but I saw the needle. No, huge didn't describe it! And he had some large vials for collection. What! I screamed to myself, so much to be taken! My doctor had the nurse put a wooden plank under the mattress and bid Me Sit up. He directed me to get into a butterfly lotus like position, and told me to hold my clasped feet tightly, while crouching my back. The doctor didn't advise me to, but as I sat there reposed like that, I prayed. Almost interrupting my prayer, the doctor instructed me to sit up. I asked him if he was no longer going to do the test and he showed me the filled vials. It was My Spinal fluid and would be sent to the labs first thing in the morning but the doctor believed without a doubt, there was nothing suspicious present. My Spinal tap was finished and I didn't even feel the initial prick of entry, I felt nothing and never knew he had started. The fluid he collected was the purest substance I had ever seen. It was like liquefied paradise. When I looked at it, I stared into an almost hypnotic pleasure. There is nothing I have ever seen, looked as pure. It is true the Lumbar test can be painful and the slightest misdirected needle can render a person crippled for life or have some other adverse neurological reaction. It became obvious to me however that under the right conditions, this very informative test can be painless.

This morning my newspaper man, actually My Sister's paper I collect around 6:00 a.m., told me he was going for an operation to the spine. He said he would be convalescing for about 6 weeks and made provisions to have someone bring the paper. I wished him well and said a silent prayer as he drove away. It was this that set me thinking of spinal tests and remembering the purity of healthy spinal fluid. The more I think of this fluid, the easier it is to accept how wondrous our bodies truly are. Even and especially at the microscopic level, the simple stem cells contain genetic codes capable of enormous feats, impossible to simulate by man. We are only now starting to understand these simple cells. Imagine the complexity of comprehending how this whole body works. Our healthy condition can change in the blink of an eye but I believe the reverse is also true. We might experience change for the better and with a similar blink, can wipe away diseases that long presented problems. Cures may only be a breath away and treatment is constantly evolving.

Imagine the painless Lumbar Tap, Spinal Surgery and all the medical procedures impossible a generation ago.

We do not know our time but what time we have, even a simple moment, can do wondrous things. A moment's gesture Might Spread like the ripple in a lake, moving away from a single dropped pebble and might reach the banks. Your smile can carry MileS away. Kind words may be curative for plaguing stress. Sometimes the smallest gesture packs the biggest punch and even a "Huge" needle in a spinal tap can be painless

Crying wolf

For the entire season the famed Dr. House misdiagnosed almost every other patient with having MS. I call it the Misdiagnosis Season. It is very difficult to watch the kinds of symptoms that might manifest themselves and be signals for MS. Furthermore, to have to deal with the possibility of any visiting you. Perhaps one of the more unsettling episodes on the show for me was with the guest appearance of Rap Artist turned actor, reputable family man, exercise guru and referred to by a fellow celeb as Luscious Lips, Mr. LL Cool J.

In 2005 the TV series House M.D, Season 2 Episode 1, dubbed Appearance, LL Cool J played the role of an inmate on death row who was having some very unusual symptoms which left the doctors guessing or up in arms. I had been recently diagnosed and wasn't yet coming to grips with or understanding what MS was. Watching Dr. House was supposed to be casual pastime but I was growingly disturbed by the Many Symptoms the great Dr. House thought were associated with MS. He was on his traditional whiteboard as he eliminated what the illnesses weren't and almost every time, the most frightening symptoms were still potential telltales for MS.

When I saw LL Cool J battling with electrical shocks through his body which threw him into uncontrollable seizures, it was getting all too familiar and the doctor's words that the illness manifests itself differently in all patients were starting to seem too much like the "crossed-eyed" shooting at clay pigeons. I learned of the debilitating way the illness strikes but had never associated pain, severe pain with it. I was wrong, not only did Dr. House suggest it but some very gripping pains confirmed pain was going to be a part of this illness. The Philippian doctor that visited my hospital bed would have been well served to have watched any episode of House M.D and perhaps would not have been so dismissing of my complaints.

The waiting for the next symptom was too overwhelming and prayers invited me to research my illness. My vision was too impaired to read print and the monitor on the computer never stayed quiet long enough for me to focus, it kept pulsing in and out even when the colors had returned. My Sister is very au fait with research and has particular prowess in digital searches. Her equal curiosity and deep desire to put us both at ease through knowing what to expect and do, compelled her to delve into the intricacies of MS. She was my initial source of all things to do and on doctor's visits, acted as my ears and eyes. Through her, we established my routines, especially my diet. Had not for her, many of the doctors' words would have been lost in My Scattered thoughts, as I visited. She remained focused and had great recall of detail. I fervently endorse having someone accompany you to the doctors and if you are as fortunate as I was, your companion would absorb all you couldn't handle. For years I went with friends on visits but I was thinking only to be supportive and never realized how vital listening and recalling would eventually prove to be.

Today, I am now schooled in my illness and I have experienced a diverse onslaught of its symptoms. My education warns me of the impending dangers and close association with other patients has prepared me for likely episodes of MS. My body will be ravaged by MS in ways hard to imagine and treatment is as sketchy as the Abominable Snowman. I welcome all new ideas of treating this illness but I am very aware that what might work for some, doesn't work for all. Due to the diverse episodic manifestations of the illness and the vastness of its intrusion on the body, I imagine that many proposed cures might only work on a cross section of cases. Of course, the unscrupulous vultures that prey on the weak and destitute will also offer their "snake oils" to those desperately seeking an end to their torment, one other than death. I too want to find that Miracle Solution to vanquish this invasive enemy. I can assure you it's not crying wolf when we scream for help. The day presents many reasons to scream but we choose carefully when to bid someone to come running.

The Lord My Savior has made my experiences with this illness much more tolerable and inspires me to use what time I have, reminding me, He alone knows the time and date and my doctors are shooting blindly but with His blessings can serve me.

My fight is not to balance on my feet, or see your face, I understand my limitations. My daily fight is to feed the good wolf inside of me, to nurture it with wholesomeness and the righteous breads. The old Indian told his grandson of the two wolves within man, the evil and the good. He explained that the one who is fed the most is the stronger and in defeating the other, will dominate the person. If you feed the evil wolf with its breads of hatred, anger, doubts, fears, deceitfulness and the like, it suppresses the good wolf. Its growls and snarls become evident as its strength continues to grow. The good wolf thrives on a smile, a soft word, sincerity, warmth, kindness and other breads of love. Give us this day our daily bread.

When Love stops liking

She was the fastest in the neighborhood and defeated both boys and girls our age

and size groups. We shared a mutual affinity for each other and those preteen

days were full of adventure. I moved out of Deacons Road for years and only

returned on weekends.

During one late evening when the local boys, you know wild boys, met, there was a

speed competition to see who was the fastest around our connecting gaps. Rose was

the reigning champion but the guys wanted me, "Buddy over street" to challenge

her. Some of you might remember where I got that nickname, you might even recall

the opening theme narration from the TV series "Run Buddy Run," way back in the

late 60's. Maybe the Merrymen's "Run Buddy Boy" was inspired by it. I think I can

still hear the narrator, "This is Buddy Overstreet. He is wanted by the head of the

most powerful crime syndicate in the country. In a steam room Buddy overheard

their vital secrets and the mysterious words Chicken Little. Now he knows too

much. These are the orders given to all members of the syndicate from one end of

the country to the other. Get Him! Get Him! Get Him!"

Buddy was constantly on the run, moving and escaping his pursuers by a hair. The guys at school thought I was fast on the street, out walking everyone and ducking through cars. So at Wesley Hall, some called me Buddy Over Street, others just stuck to Johnson baby powder.

They pitted me against My Secret sweetheart. We stood back to back, awaited their "Ready, set go!" and were off in opposite directions around the circular gaps. We met on the blind side of the gaps and crossed each other at the approximate midpoint. In meant the race was tied to that point but my noble sweetheart must have deliberately slowed down on the return home because I broke the finish first and knew I was far too winded to finish ahead of her when she looked so unspent. The guys in their undeveloped male chauvinism, applauded me in celebration of the ill-perceived gender dominance. I defeated the champion but I knew in my heart, I never accomplished their desired feat.

Looking back over the years, I wonder what other successes I achieved because others nobler forfeited. Who else stepped aside that I might step in? Who stepped down that I can step up? There can be no good unless there is bad or rich unless there is poor. When I won, someone lost. The feeling of achievement is great but there is agony in defeat. How then do I justify celebrations when someone else is heartbroken by insufficiency? I am not sure people like winners who brazenly taunt the losers. My competitive spirit, whenever there was "One on one," became very flawed and although I showed commendable skills in games like table tennis and chess, it was too daunting to win. I therefore made a terrible competitive player but aside from matches, I did well.

My team mates applauded My Skills but were often frustrated by my lack lustered performance when faced with a singular opponent. It was this inefficiency of the "Eye of the Tiger" that kept me away from competing in "One on one" sports. My friends never truly understood why the guy who could face the biggest bullies was timid in "One and one" competition but good for me, they never could. I might have been seen in an even worse light if they knew I was battling with an emotional conflict.

I am therefore no stranger to conflicts of the mind and body, so when MS struck, I knew it was me against my body, a "One on one" battle again. I knew I was faced with that demon that plagued my life. This time, I was determined to not let my competition win. I didn't want to have My Spectators frustrated by my inefficiency to fight back. I could not roll over to its cruelty and have it do its worse. But, I don't have the "Eye of the Tiger." It never developed. Those looking on never see my war paint but they do see the results of my battle. Family Might See me curl to the blows but I refuse to take a ten count, lying on the canvas. I rise up and clap my gloves and make ready for the next episode. My opponent tackles with a cowardice that masquerades in an obscurity to prevent the medical fraternity from tracking its movements. Consequently it is illusive, but it is real and it solicits the help of my own nerves, which like traitors, work against me. This mutiny concocted by my enemy would have taken the battle from me very early had I not solicited help of my own. Remember, "One on one" I was never a true performer but within me there was the skill. When I learned that MS took over my nerves and stopped their functioning or caused them to fire ghost impulses; have me experience what was not my reality, I decided MS can take My Senses but not My Soul, My System but not My Spirit. It was no longer "One on one," I solicited the help of the

Almighty and with the prayers and support of My Spectators, I am cheered to the finishing line, there is no blind side on this track. MS will not forfeit as did My Sweetheart in childhood. I have to race to the end and although I feel winded, I am fueled with a strength that is more powerful in times of weakness and I press on.

When some of my friends learned of my illness they smiled and said Johnno does get ill. They were true to a point, I was their superman and never took time away from school or work for illness, so I always had the perfect record of attendance. But I met my krypton. Some who loved before, can't look on at me now because of my lifestyle change. They have trouble coming to grips with a Johnno who can no longer run that lap, or face up to the bullies. In their minds' eye, they do not want to see a broken bodied me. They probably still love me but don't like what they now know and see. I no longer hide with emotional conflicts, it is important that I give my all. This battle requires every aspect of me and in particular, Mental Stability. MS plays Mock Sport with the body and May Sometimes convince you that you are in a different reality. You walk into a room that has normal ambience yet perceive it to be a flaring furnace. Nothing around you burns yet about you, it is as hot as raw flames. I guess it is hard for your love ones to look on and see you face with an invisible enemy. They can't possibly like what you are now faced with and sometimes their emotion conflict. They wish they could come around and spend quiet moments with you but in their minds' eyes, the image of you past and you present tears them apart. They don't like what they see and you understand. I don't like what I face either but my furnace is unreal just as the conception of what you Might See in me. If you look closely, I hope you see what I now feel. My Strength beyond the brute force that over powered the bullies. My Strength that battles the invisible enemy and lifts me up to fight again tomorrow. If we allow our minds to overpower our hearts then our battles have already been lost. The fuel that sustains me is the energies of those who fight back their feelings long enough to not let dislike get in the way. When love stops liking we will never achieve real goals and successfully battle our demons.

I walk bent and labored but I lift up my eyes in the face of my new bully. My fight is no longer muscles and snarls but spiritual health and quiet prayer. I will run to the finish line with exuberance because unlike My Sweetheart, MS will not forfeit from affection but rather, hopes to stop me with affliction.

Emancipated from MySelf

A compulsion to give my all and do my best led me into a marriage that died a bitter end.

From day one I was determined to show my worth and worked at it the moment I stepped into the door. It was an unusually long meeting that resulted in Me Speaking of things I hadn't for years. But I was relaxed. She was playfully smiling and basically gave me her approval. She bid me return, ready for work the following week, which was a matter of a weekend away. I didn't know the celebrations with my family that evening were leading to a road of bondage, without the ball and chain.

I showed up for work on Monday morning and was there through Saturday. The job meant giving up hockey practice early Saturday mornings and that disqualified me from the lustrous field life, having played center forward for the school team since I was merely 12 years old. It also signaled the end to the social life I knew. Slowly it pulled me in and banished me from the extracurricular thing I loved dearly. Losing this love perhaps made me a bit cold to other loves and opened me to fall further slave to the mistress that took my all.

My devotion to the job saw me working non-stop during the day with brief breaks for lunch but later no lunch. I was rewarded with promotions and new responsibilities and in little time, was managing the largest Retail business of its kind on the island and as I learned later, throughout the Caribbean. My devotion to my quasi wife united me to an allegiance to our children, almost 30 staff and soon the union took me completely. I was slave to my compulsion to give my all, and took little time away. The job grew larger and eventually we installed branches in new areas. They thrived better than the other failed, similar businesses in the areas and remained viable undertakings for years. But My Skills led to further promotions and soon, perhaps too big. My ideas for further growth never stopped but my immediate bosses didn't want to experiment with the kinds of change I recommended and with changing time, the digital age overcame us.

I was lured away for two years by a new mistress and then lured back. Wanting to be even More Successful with the new encouragements and incentives, I started to work on Sundays. With absolutely no social life now, it was easy to pursue the invitation of one of my clients and show up for a Sunday meeting at the Gymnasium. I asked my way around the Complex and was directed to a room where they introduced me to ballroom dancing. This was going to be my only outing and since it was on Sundays after my working hours, I decided, why not. It was incredible how the husband and wife team Leon and Camilla, were able to organize this dance studio, called Genesis and for me it was truly a genesis. I showed up every Sunday, never missing one. I adjourned work many Sundays and went directly to the Studio. After successfully taking my first practical exams in dance, I had found a new life. The dance floor became an escape from the stress of my working day and I was there during the week as well. They taught us Latin, Ballroom and Line dancing, all beyond fun. It was like a new paradise. My Social skills were rusty and my anomic aphasia doesn't allow me to recall the names of many of those who made the escape so magnetic.

But, it met an abrupt end. The paradise that kept me away from my mistress was going to be snatched away from me. My feet were first to protest and tingling in my toes with increasing sensation of numbness were rude warnings that all was not well. The numbness first seemed like I was wearing socks up to my ankles but later the socks climbed beyond my knees and were in the middle of my thighs. Mobility was unsteady and my vision to the right doubled. A very close friend assisted me up and down the stairs at work until she insisted she take me to seek help. Stacey drove me in my car to the doctor's from work one morning and when I was admitted to private hospital, I watched her driving away that night. It's been over 10 years now that I have driven a car, danced to a Salsa or Waltz. I miss the social life at the Dance Studio and also my friends there. A visit from Leon and Camilla recently brought back a flood of good memories and the role they played in paving that escape from stress.

Last night when going to bed and using the quiet time to count my blessings, I wanted to count my friends at dancing and recall the memories. They were too many good ones again and it was keeping me awake rather than lulling me to sleep. Together the group with the cruise trips, picnics, Balls, exhibitions, parties and still more, made it easy to enjoy my aging process and have a life, a real life. I watch TV shows with dancing like "So you think you can dance" and my body feels to move but I can't even tap rhythmically with my feet. I tried to follow games like field hockey and tennis on the screen but the ball disappears and the games make little sense. It is increasingly difficult to watch life disappear and gradually it becomes easier to reflect on the memories. Every moment has magic and recalling them is to live them.

MS robbed me of living that paradise but the bonds of friendship withstood the changing times and I enjoy the lasting memories I recall, in quiet time as I prepare to rest at night.

Once again, there is no stress and I am emancipated from MySelf

84

On the threshold of change

I was called to her office and told my conduct at work was exemplary. She had observed me for a week after she returned from her vacation, just two weeks after I got the job. It was to express her intension to transfer me to a more challenging role. Fresh out of military and school training, some things were so deeply imbedded, they came out spontaneously, just like my "Thank you mam!" did. She would have none of it and compliments quickly changed into accusations of rudeness. Conflicted by a new awareness that "mam" was rude, I bowed my head in shame and humbleness. To offer further respect, I did as I was taught and never looked My Senior in the eyes. My humble stance served only to frustrate my accuser more, "Look at me when I am speaking to you!" she reprimanded, and as I stood, torn between disciplines, I was lost. I was never labelled disobedient or rude and there in that instance, I couldn't seem to step away from this conduct. I tried to remain quiet and not put my foot further in. I took My Scolding. Dismissed, I politely stepped back, caught the doorknob and apologized as I turned it, but I said, "I'm sorry mam!" There was that "mam" again, it came out without me thinking and when I heard my blunder, I apologized for it profusely, "So sorry mam!" and

86

again there was a "mam." I was hopeless and she was so frustrated she said, "Just

go!"

Schooling and the military drilled the "mams" and "sirs" in so tightly, they were

difficult, near impossible to dislodge. The change was not easy. In fact, change

with any of the things that became intrinsic, proved difficult as time went on.

Losing friends for whatever reason always resulted in change, change that I have

not yet mastered. Reflecting on those I lost to death during this year alone, in a

weak way, I still imagine they are out there, somewhere, and one day I might come

across them. Not being able to experience closure by dressing and going to

funerals has left me in limbo and the notice of their untimely deaths has not sunk

in. It is like they are just as scarce as they had always been.

When I explain to inquirers about not being able to dress in socially acceptable

wear for occasions other than the very casual, they never fully appreciate what

effect it has on my life. The imprisonment I feel in my own home and the unintended banishment from society is perhaps an even greater change than adjusting to this frail body.

Tonight many will make resolutions and vows to close the doors on things old as they ring in things new. Relationships will be forged with the conviction to embrace change in their lives. Years ago, I made resolutions of my own. Doors I slammed close behind me and I looked forward to opening new ones. In 2004, I started to experience change just as the year turned. Not what I had hoped for but change that later forced me to close the doors to My Social and professional lives. Every year since then, almost like clockwork, there have been major changes in my health. It would be great if these changes had been improvements but no change has improved any of the old conditions. I get used to a new state during the year and as changes step in, adjustments are made.

I slammed shut the doors to anger, to hatred and worry and have thrown the keys so far away, I could never find them. Some things I left behind with no hopes of turning back and some new ones I found with no intensions to lose them.

Through all the changing, the physical and emotional adjustments, one positive change I experience is a growing spiritual health with an increasing faith in God and the work He intends for us. I listen to many chastise His works and apparent lack of participation in their lives and I remember the times it seemed like He wasn't hearing me either. That eventually changed and I hope it will be one of your changes. Whatever lies ahead, I am more prepared to face it now than I had ever been. We know that change awaits us but we don't know what it will bring. Sometimes it's hard to close the door on things you got used to but in order to move on, to drive forward, we can't look back. What I do know is that nothing is mightier than the love of God. I could never fight my battles alone and with Him I shall never be alone. With Him, I found you. It was His love that brought you in my life. Your role, however insignificant you think it is or was, has helped move the mountains that laid before me. My Story, should it be told, is a sad one but it has a happy ending. I share glimpses into its intricacies but I am guarded with some more telling specifics because they might uncover private moments I have no right disclosing that involve the lives of others who share precious time with me.

In the end love diminishes the pain and overcomes the suffering. Love triumphs and has been the one change I will usher in and wish for you. It is true love that conquers all and I have true love. The love and appreciation for life, family and friends. This love is mightier than all things. If it sounds familiar, it should be!

This coming year and the years ahead, I hope and pray that the worse is behind you and that true prosperity is within your grasp. Embrace change. Love!

Have a Happy New Year!

Knock, Knock, Knocking on Heavens door.

They told me the medication was going to be costly. I had lost my job and had no means to sustain life if it was going to be dependent on this drug from the German company Bayer, with a spelling Betazeron but somehow written and sounded Betaferon. I did my due diligence and read up on this drug, only to find out cost was going to be the least of my worries. Case studies had shown the side effects were frightening and many users stop because of the repeated torment. The doctors suggested I be trained in its use if I wanted to forego the high cost to have it administered. As if the $300.00 tag for dosage wasn't enough for the every other day medication, I would need to pay a nurse $50.00 to administer My Subcutaneous injections. The more I read, the greater my reluctance. On my final visit, my private doctor advised the drug would not cure but it would stave off episodes of MS considerably and slow its debilitative hold on my body. He told me I should consider the public hospital for my continual treatment since cost was going to be burdensome, especially since there was no real income.

It was clear I had little choice but to heed his advice. I remember him telling me once, there was nothing further the medical fraternity could do to help and if I were a believer, I should pray. How could you not trust a doctor such as him? I had been praying all along and I received the prayers of church groups, friends and family. My sister's and mother's prayer meets every evening, were unaware to me during the first year. They were retiring to their rooms at the same time each evening and folk from other homes were doing the same. They collectively screamed for my help. The Lord must have answered because, I had no fear and I developed a great understanding of what was happening to my body. I became so aware that doctors brought their touring firms to listen to me present. I watched student doctors look on with amazement and received the compliments of their lead doctors.

I decided to take the medication and halt or slow the onslaught and uncertainty of the episodes. But if I were going to be injecting my body with this highly toxic drug, I needed to pray intensively for protection against its ravages. I lost the natural and fluid use of my body, but I didn't want to lose my cognitive sense. I remember the feeling during seizures, of an inability to piece together simple sentences while I was unconscious. I remember fighting in my mind to make just three words into a sentence and couldn't get it done, for what seemed like hours but in reality was only 20 seconds of unconsciousness. I prayed many days before getting the medication and each time before taking it.

Whispers told me to scrub up surgically before every injection and my mother and I ensured very sanitary preparations. I read of the dangers of needle site infections and how the medication burns holes in these sites. I knew more and more the importance of my prayers. Once you got started on the medication, stopping would be detrimental to my wellbeing and the quality of life, if there was life, would be greatly reduced. You may think of it like the medication is a dam that prevents episodes from flooding the body and allows only trickles of them to seep through its walls. If the medication is removed for only a short period of time, the episodes will escape and gush to overwhelm the body. That being the case, we needed to operate with great efficiency to Make Sure we get the every other days perfectly organized and to never miss a day. It was also very important to administer as close to the same time each day, to be hours late was to shake the dam and cause larger cracks, to be too early was to overdose. I keep a journal to record every injection, where and when taken, to ensure greater accuracy. My doctor marvels at the condition of my thorax and thighs, the absence of injection site problems.

I have been a good patient using this medication every other day since March 2006, however, this holiday season, I was held hostage and could receive no medication from the hospital. My fight to remedy the impasse failed and on Christmas Eve I was given the bad news that there was no medication available for me. I knew there was no likelihood of receiving any on Christmas Day when I was due and since Friday was a holiday and the suppliers were close on weekends, there was no hope of getting the medication before Monday. This would mean taking the dam down for 5 days, missing 2 days of medication. It was with that notice that I retired to my room with earnest prayers. I needed a miracle and for the Lord to be like that dam and protect me from the rigors of the piling episodes. I keep saying episodes with no clarity. The episodes are things symptomatic with MS and for me I had the blindness in alternate eyes, the unsteadiness in mobility with easy imbalance. What I describe as the "Truck" was a period of 15 to 30 seconds of feeling like something squashing my hand. I had roaming hot patches which was like a hot iron pressing against an area on the body, somewhat like branding cattle. It went on for about 10 seconds and recurred every 20 minutes over a 3 weeks period then migrated to another area. The list goes on. Imagine the anticipation of these episodes bursting through and overwhelming me, possibly all at once. Imagine waking up to darkness which remains pitch black even after lights are turned on. Imagine trying to climb out of bed but having no support and buckling on your feet. Nerves control everything and one of my episodes was the tightening of My Skin and organs after light touches. A shower meant the contracting of my lungs and heart from the gentle spray. They seemed no end to what I might expect.

On Christmas Eve when I prayed, I later got a whisper that told me I was supposed to do something in about 7 days. In order to do this I would need be well. That I believed was the affirmation I would not be battered by the threatening episodes. I wasn't to go "Knock, knock, knocking on Heaven's door." I reassured a friend who had been very worried, that all was going to be well and I was able to say it with certainty.

Yesterday I got my medication at around 6:00 pm and apart from a bit more instability in my legs and a weird sensation in my head, I was ok and here a few hours later, I am back to my normal. I feel rather strongly about government, hospital administrators and suppliers all having this influence on my quality of life and I continue to pray for God's guidance of these men in control. I am not just a case and statistic, and I believe I still can play a role in society and should not be counted out and treated with such a perceived lack of urgency and priority. However, MS - Mighty Spirit, My Soul and My Strength is in My Saviour. Once again the Lord has answered my earnest prayers and delivered me out of the clutches of this Menacing Sickness, MS.

Makes you forget

The symptoms of MS can be cruel and unforgiving. Can take away your physical and mental health, anything nerve related, as quickly as the blink of an eye. It is unpredictable and you can spend conscious moments worrying which nerve is next affected. Would it be the nerves that coordinate the gentle waves of your respiration or the rhythmic beats of your heart? What about the timely control of your bladder? It's no wonder so many afflicted go insane, if it's not your loss of the abilities that gets you, the worries of what's next might.

The nerves that control the upkeep of my memory centre have not been affected and I thrive on recalling times etched in my heart. Childhood memories that could easily have escaped me but helped to the surface by visual reminders of chief actors that played leading roles. I was watching a show recently where kids were asked to say a memory they hold dearest of their dad. Their dad is a huge celebrity and each reminisced of their childhood. I couldn't quite understand how it is that someone so dear to his public, who speaks so lovingly of his family, is remembered by his adult children for the childhood past and in very specific deeds. I tried to find that one deed, I might have chosen if placed in the same situation but it was troubling to limit choices, hard to find a single time frame to represent the man who played his role so memorably.

I do have early childhood memories and the ones Most Standing out are the outings to the pasture and the beach. Almost everywhere we went, my dad encouraged healthy competition. We used to run from the top of the hill, touch the mile trees at the bottom and run back to daddy. I was just over knee high when it started and was beaten by both my older siblings each time. Cherie would sometimes stop for me and encourage me to press on. Perhaps that was when the bond started growing and why we became so close later. Daddy took us to the beach and taught us to hold our breath and made us less afraid of the water. I have flashes of our beach times and the memories frozen in pictures that my dad took for my Mom Since she was abroad studying and wasn't there to watch us mature to teens. He played the mommy and daddy roles at home for many of our formative years and since it was not his intention to do every task, encouraged us to learn to take care of our own laundry; there were no washing machines, just hand wash. We experimented in the kitchen and learned to cook and bake from very early too. He never baked cakes but we loved anything he cooked. He stopped cooking when mommy returned home after seven years of studies, but pitched in if it became necessary. Daddy was a one pot kind of cook but mommy did all kinds of things. She introduced us the fried rice, casserole pies, tossed salads, chow mein, lasagna and other delicacies we enjoyed. Her work load and eventual back troubles from it, prevented her enjoying the hours of meals preparation and cooking became a burden. My dad was like her knight in shining armor and saw to her every need just as he did ours. He became the dominant cook in the house and soon we were back to his chicken down in rice, cook-ups, cou cou, soups and rice 'n stews. They were all very tasty, never looked like they could taste like anything, especially following the colorful dishes from mommy, but were remarkably tasty. So much so that when we had guests from overseas, he took care of the cooking. His jug jug should have won national acclaim and international too, judging from the many family members who came from overseas Christmas time looking forward to it.

My dad was a celebrity of sorts. His confectionery van pulling up in the school yards was always to the joy of students. He sold sweets to the canteens and always gave me a pocket full to take to the kids. They always fantasized what it was like being me, having the sweetie man as your dad, and found it hard to understand why I was never as into sweets as they were. Dad later became the whisky man and I went along with him on occasions too. The men's faces always lit up like the kids from school. Dominoes slamming and salutations above the slams were routed to my dad. They seemed to love him even more that the children and more dependent on their sweets too. We went to his cricket games when we were very young but were too caught up with children's play to notice his achievements. Later, when we were old enough to pay some attention, we noticed his face adorned the walls of his cricket clubs and he had pictures of presentations of awards from Governor Generals. My dad was the cricketer extraordinaire, whose batting and bowling skills earned him great accolades in every local club. When he wasn't making runs for them he was scoring against them or bowling them out. I heard many of the club stories of the ease with which he blasted sixes and some of them were so stunning, they seemed unreal. But they were true. My dad played illustrious cricket even into his early 60's. My game was hockey and when I visited a club and they heard the name, I became Johnno's son.

After I left school I went on an interview at my father's work place and although my qualifications spoke for themselves our shared name spoke more highly for me. I was always Adrian Johnson Jr. That was my name, we answered the phone at home junior or senior but being Adrian Johnson meant living up to the accolades bestowed on my dad. To his public he was the greatest salesman and cricketer, a charmer of the ladies and got along with all people. My dad was all these and much more to me, I could never compete. I didn't have the skills to be a great salesman, I could only sell your needs and was too honest to encourage your wants. My cricketing skills were good but I didn't have a love for playing its long version, waiting almost a month of weekends for the completion of one game. I like field hockey were we could go home with the glory within the hour of play. Although I get along with most people, I cannot socialize with drunks and chimneys. I can't watch sorrows being drown and good health abused or opportunity lost from discouraging buddies. The charming trait, common to the Johnson Males Skipped me, it seemed you needed to lie to gain favor and boast of exploits to harness respect. I wanted them both but not if it meant corrupting our integrity. I took my dad's name but it looked like I wouldn't get his fame.

He raised us kids with a rigidness that made us all ready to step up to responsibility and we all did, for most of our lives anyway. We saw his loyalty and strength. For us our dad was unbreakable but when we saw him cry like a child for the first time ever, at his mother's funeral, we saw the sensitive frailty that was protected these years by his harsh exterior. We never heard even a hint that there was a soft side to our dad until then. It must have always been there but it was guarded with layers that never yielded to the battering of four children as he raise us alone. We respected our dad deeply and even when I was promoted to Manager in the company and he was still a van salesman for liquors and sweets, I was still humbled by his path.

While in a training with other managers, we were asked to each say who we respected the most and why. I listened as the circle of people got closer to me and one after the other, they said the same thing. Each respected their department's director. I respected mine too but when it came time for me to make My Submissions, the man I respected the most was my dad. There at the same company with his lowly job and on his own for seven years with four children, he managed to raise us all to be heads in our schools, provided contented lives for us, protected us from peer pressure and did it all while becoming, the best at all things, be it work, cricket or parenting. Apart from all that, my dad can step into a rum shop to the applause of bibbers, walk on to a cricket pitch with praises and go to a dress up staff party and get the admiration of many for his candor.

I saw him cry again when I got ill. He cried every time he started to talk to anyone about my illness and on one of my visits to the doctor when I relayed to him their intention to keep me for tests, he cried again. Tears seemed constant from this tower of strength and it seemed to take a toll on him. His outer shell soon matched his frail interior. In the space of a few years, he went from his broad shouldered 200 Lbs. to a bent scary frame of 156 Lbs. For months of my illness, he assisted me with My Showers and made my every meal for the first three years. He took me on every car trip and sat with me on mornings for hours before setting out. I saw his dwindling form and heard a wavering tone in his voice whenever he discussed my illness. The first two years, I spent his birthdays in the hospital so when I was at home the third year, he came out hugged me and said how happy he was to be able to celebrate his day with me at home. How great it was to have me here. My dad took on a new persona during my early illness, the first years broke his spirit and soon later he was a ghost of himself.

Today, I can't recognize him. Not only is he a frailer man, he has become bitter and seems to have no confidence in anyone or anything. I don't believe it should be attributed to my illness but if it is, then MS has taken a far greater toll on my family than on me.

She was only 16

She was very young when she started getting her kids. I was the third of four and was only 8 months in the womb when my parents finally tied the knot. You Might Say, I was her only child to attend the wedding and we wore the gown perfectly.

They cut the umbilical cord that bonded us closely for the gestating 9 months, just 23 days before she celebrated her 20th birthday. Today she celebrates yet another birthday, notice I didn't say which because I am oblige to observe a female desire to have you guess. Looking on at her for countless years she passed as a sibling to her kids.

She left to study nursing in England when I was 5 and returned to find me, a head strong teenager, who adored her very presence. I wasn't a mother's boy but I worked closely with her, having been assigned kitchen duties from when I was 8 years old. It placed me by her side when she baked and cooked. My mom returned to Barbados with a smashing figure. I still can close my eyes and see the Hollywood image of my dad running across the airport floors to catch her and sweep her off her feet, twirl and kiss. They were like young lovers and that played out for the better part of my life. Their love and commitment raised us 4 kids and even with their modest means, they overcame many financial challenges and we never felt the constraints of poverty.

I watched my mom worked Monstrous Shifts, sometimes leaving for work at 9:00 p.m. returning at 7:00 a.m. and back off to work after only a few hours, to do a Midday Shift. She was very devoted to nursing and after her retirement was invited to return as a consultant in the Neo-Natal ward where she had spent her final years at the hospital. Some years afterwards when the burden had become too much on her feet and back, apparent wounds of nursing, she retired from hospital duties, but in a few years later, assumed a new role of private nurse to me. My illness requires constant attention and medication must be like clockwork, administered in a very sterile environment. The kitchen duties of preparing my meals demand a careful watch on diet, which must be kept with little variation. Sometimes her natural flair wants to color my bland meals but medication prohibits even green leafy veggies, citrus fruit and too much Vitamins C or K. Imagine, I shouldn't even drink mauby, a favorite. She is like a watch dog, checking all labels before acquiring products when out shopping. My impaired vision prevents double scrutiny so again, I am as attached to her as with the umbilical cord.

The years are now taking their toll on her and neither of us can hide the signs of aging. Yet, despite her personal medical challenges she still treats me with priority. She is no longer sharp witted and we differ in our attitudes about many things in life but, love is never lost and our frail bodies are masked with strengthening spirits. Many of us reflect on our mother's role in our growing years but I have a distinct pleasure of being close to my mother all through my life.

I rushed out to the mail man every day when she was away studying with hopes of mail coming from England. She speaks of taking me into town as a toddler and having Me Sing to the workers. I recall fashioning my letters to look like hers on paper because it made me feel a piece of her while at school. We played table tennis on the dining table when she returned and while she and I played scrabble in the bunk bed one day, I jumped down to again catch the postman for expected mail from England and he had it. Her results came from the qualifying examinations and together we celebrated the newly awarded Register Nurse.

It was my mom that took me to Combermere on mornings and who waited for me on evenings. She attended Many School functions and even became familiar with some of my buddies. The decades of admiration and adoration cannot be condensed into text, short enough to read and still give the kind of credit she deserves. These last few years my mom watched her baby, though a Man, Stumbling and learning to walk all over. She bought the sketch pads and pencils to help Me Sketch again and commended My Scrawls. I saw her face when she had all but given up, when I laid attached to machines and tubes. Her grown man was a baby again and required similar attention back down to bathing and feeding.

I am now beyond that dependence but still have not become fully independent and she is there when I need her. We don't know the minds of others but we can know their hearts and my mother's heart has always been with me and My Siblings. We have much to be thankful for in her and lots to admire from this 16 years old girl who raise 4 kids in spite of great challenges and has now become a grandmother

and great grandmother, times over.

I wish my mother a very Blessed Birthday, with lots and lots of love, appreciation

and adoration!

Sharing the Nativity

My Sister came over and decorated a corner of the room with a nativity set which she pieced together over years and have now painted them into a Matching Set. They look like they came boxed together.

I regret that I can't get to see them like you could and regret that my camera can't capture them like the naked eye but either way, this glimpse reminds me why we abandoned a tree and have clung to the nativity.

The setting tells the story and seems to propel my thoughts back in time when this king of king and lord of lords was born to bring peace to all men. I feel the peace and want very much to share this peace with my friends. Perhaps the picture can tell the thousand words they say it can and maybe you would feel the peace and goodwill I feel each time I look at it.

Hope you can enjoy the rest of this Yule Tide and that you experience the reason

for the season. Spread the love my friends

So this is Christmas

I played Santa Claus years ago. Not with the suit, just the presents. It was my joy to show up long before others arrived, leave gifts in plain sight then pretend I was as shock as they were to find them. What a pleasure it was to watch their unsuspecting faces, full of glee for the simplest token of good wishes, during this time of the year.

Like thousands of Bajans, I waited to the last minute to shop in the hustle and bustle, largely because I worked retail all of my professional life and had to be present during store hours. There was another reason though, I loved to stumble across old faces long erased from My Shallow recall and the rush time seemed best to see them. Quick hellos, joyous greetings for the holidays followed by wishes of prosperity for the coming year and off we rushed without the need of excuses.

From a boy, Christmas Meant Sea sand and rocks paving the walk ways, snow on the mountain trees, manicured hedges, dried sorrel, varnished floors, new furniture or the old made to look new, English apples, red imported grapes, Falernum, Kola

Tonic, Jug Jug, the aroma of freshly baked ham and cakes - great cake especially, lots of cleaning, dressing the Christmas tree and the anticipation of gifts. Yeah, what's in my box?

Many of these things are still part of Christmas for you but for me and by your reasoning, My Season has become drab. I go nowhere, buy no gifts, and cannot enjoy the eats and drinks I once clamored for. In fact, I am not even sure my voice will allow me to speak and for sure, I long lost the ability to sing, so no caroling. Playing the flute, saxophone or violin is no longer a doable choice at any time, and so not during the season.

Christmas has taken a new complexion for me. The people around all look so happy but they are sad reminders of things I miss the most. What used to be the most joyous time of the year has become MS - My Saddest

Watching others do the work is no fun and in reality, it is painful to not be a part of the dress up and preparations. Perhaps if the memories of past Christmases had been eroded like my dexterity and senses, I would not be as sad during the season.

But yet, amidst the missing of the things that meant Christmas, there is a peace that spreads through me. It could be that this is the "Peace and Goodwill," I had been wished by friends like you, all my life. It could otherwise be that this is what Christmas is really about, MS - My Sense of contentment. No need for rushing or overworking. It could be the opportunity to spread good cheer without having to wrap it. The remodeling of oneself and not the fixing up of exteriors and the superficial sprucing of houses and rooms. It could also be a retrospection of the year gone and the inspection of the road ahead. It could be wishes that have earnest sincerity for good health and prosperity and not just the fleeting salutations I once shared as we bumped into each other while we shopped.

Friends, forgive me that I no longer follow the course of tradition and that I breach the routines of Christmas. I know my past Christmases and I enjoyed them with you. I hope that my absence of gifts giving and those unscheduled, surprise meetings or the casual wishes of merriment, serve to alert you that I am now in a different place where tangible gifts pleasure only the surface and that your spirit of honesty and kindness is valued beyond all riches. Know friend that warm words now embrace more than your arms, which could actually be physically painful due to my tactile nerve malfunction. "I have no gifts to bring," was the drummer boy's call and is now mine. But take my earnest appreciation and sincerest wishes for a Blessed Christmas and a Prosperous New Year!

I don't get to live my old Christmases but these Christmases, I live. So this is Christmas!

http://bit.ly/JohnnoBim

Our School song says it all

My Siblings all went to St. Leonard's school, as did our parents. It was not the most welcoming news to hear I had passed for Combermere and I felt some mixed emotions. I heard lots of negative undertones as my family described life at the "High School." I was predestined to fail in their untested subjects like Latin, Physics and Chemistry and my preconception of the others was dismal. I sat through classes with the haunt of doom in my early life but sitting with my classmates, I felt no trepidation. In fact, many of them turned to "Johnson Baby Powder" for assistance.

The tradition of being slapped around the head by the senior boys was in play and juniors were certain not to venture to the top floor. My very first day at lunch was a rude awakening. The boys had crowded the canteen and I could see minimum movement of the twisted lines. With all the shouting, I marveled at how Joyce was able to hear their orders and dispatched them accurately.

After standing in line for close to 30 minutes and watching the clock's hand approach the end of lunch, I was finally 3 boys away from the counter. Morris, the school bully, barged in front of me and when I objected, "You can't do that!" he turned and said "Shut up before I cuff yah in yah mout!" I hope I got my Bajan right, I never remember if it is "uh" or "ah". I just arbitrarily interchange the spelling so that I know I am right at least half of the time. Morris turned immediately after his threat but I had to get out my protest. Still fashioned by the schooling of Sheilah Crichlow from Wesley Hall, I quite "Prim and proper" blurted out "Cuff who in whose mouth!" Actually, the word mouth never escaped my lips. My Sentence was punctuated with his brutal fist, right as promised, in the mouth. Then he turned as if he had made a clear conclusion to the dispute. Too conditioned to defend my positions, both placement in line and my feelings about what he had done, I answered him in a like manner, only, no punching. I grabbed the back of the taller bully's collar and the belt and khaki in his lower back and rammed him repeatedly to the canteen wall beneath the counter. The uproar in the canteen brought teachers running and when they parted me and were hauling me away for punishment, a crowd of strangers welcomed me with their chants and pleads to the teachers, insisting on my innocence, that I didn't start it and was only defending myself.

I got off without even a warning and received the acknowledgment of acceptance from those previously bullied and some senior boys who patted me on the back.

"Lives are in the making" at Combermere. You plant your seeds in its arable soil and in time you spring up into characters, "Ever upward to the fight" whether it be a bully or illness, whatever the circumstance. The spirit of comradery played out on that very first day and united me with a body of hundreds of souls, "Pluming wings for higher flight."

When we see wrong, we must speak up. Stand up for your right and if one man Must Sacrifice his life in the hijacked plane that all can live, if it is you, do so with focused deliberation and know that there is no greater love that this.

My friend Olivere asked why we love our Alma Mater. I love the Spirit of Combermere. The feelings of intimidation that were quelled by the support of a body of absolute strangers, the understanding of teachers who listened to the outcry of "Hungry men." I love the sense of fairness and the encouragement I received. I love that even though I had a picture painted of its old walls, following the footprints of past students through the corridors of time led me to be a stronger and braver man and shaped me into a unique individual who loves the sense of team work and loyalty. I learned these lessons in that one instance on my first day and planted these emotions in each class. I benefited from this early inoculation and through it was able to weather other storms both at school and in my life beyond.

It is MS - My Spirit, the same Combermerian spirit which made us all individuals but team players, that helps Me Soar high above the troubles which abound. My flame is bright and I face each day with all my might. I love my roots at Combermere and enjoy the fruit I now reap.

Still counting sheep?

In a movie I saw recently the protagonist advised a friend to count her blessings when she was trying to sleep and not sheep. I thought it was a novel idea but, I don't have trouble falling to sleep.

Many of my friends know I only slept 2 hours at night for all my professional life. When hospitalized, my nurses complained to the doctor that I stayed up all night listening to the television - it was only a grey audio box when I lost the perception of color and bright lights. Those 2 hours were always very sound sleep. By the time I got home and was able to use my promises box again, I got a very short promise, the first and it changed my nights ever since.

I use a magnifier to read and must have light spotted directly on the print to see it. Please don't be overly critical of my method but before I go bed at night I pray for a scripture that might have some guidance or clarity in my life. I then select the scripture randomly by letting the large print bible fall open and reading from the chapter there in. My promise is selected randomly too after a prayer for guidance. I no longer read the chapter selected, nowadays the computer reads it for me after I blindly scroll an online Bible.

That first promise was taken from Psalm 127:1, just "He giveth his beloved sleep" and that night I slept 4 hours and have slept 4 hours ever since. That is the equivalent of doubling your sleep hours and for me it is perfectly relaxing. I don't take any more than 2 minutes to fall off to sleep so there was never a need to count sheep. But that novel idea of counting my blessings was on my mind after my prayers last night and when the lights were out, I stayed there going through them.

When I started, I realize it would take too long to list them and so I started with my family. It is my parents' love that brought me to the point of proper choices and My Siblings that natured my upbringing through our close bond. I fell sleep before I could list all the reasons why my family is a blessing.

Now, instead of clearing my mind of the day's happenings, I want to go to sleep thinking of the blessings bestowed on me.

The very simple things we take for granted are blessings which if lost make life so different. Sight, the perception of color is not only about the array of prismatic refraction of light, it is about one's health and wellbeing too. The scientists have deduced from studies that green for example stimulates the eyes in a way that triggers brain cells and other body cells into a chain of restoration of health. Although the fresh air was a contributor bringing many to the island for recuperation from illnesses during the earlier years, it was the greenery that played a greater role. The countryside of lush shades of green worked at stimulating the cells so they might eliminate internal imbalances which lend to poor health. All colors play different roles on the body, you may have heard painting the inside of prisons pinky peach always tempered inmates. How ever we look at it, perception of color is a blessing, one I lost and later learned how important a colored day is.

Tonight I will count the blessings through my friendships with you.

MS – My Saviour, MS - My Sister

Before you art critics grimace disapprovingly, finding fault of my awkward stokes and imperfect eye, let me cast the first stone. I am awkward and imperfect.

I tried to come to grips with an inability to follow a line with my eyes and hands, to see pencil on white, and to focus my eyes for more than 10 seconds, without straying or blinking. I asked my mom to get me a sketching pad and dark pencils then I tried desperately to control the lead. It took hours into days before I was able to pick back up where the pencil had stopped. Making gradating shadows required varied and controlled pressure that took more time.

I started sketching after a whisper, I believed to be from MS - My Saviour. It was the same kind of whisper that guided me through difficult times so it was easy to follow. When I heard from my dear friend Asiya, she told Me Sketching was one of the therapies used on patients with MS - Multiple Sclerosis and that encouraged me to keep at it. She was right, I was able to stare without blinking for a count of 180, a remarkable achievement since I wasn't getting past 12 before. The sketch marks were becoming more obvious too and I ventured to make my rendition of the most beautiful baby picture I had ever seen.

Of course, every child is the most beautiful to its parents but this is not my child. There is a bias however, this is my baby sister who turns 50 today.

Alana was transferred to the third form in Combermere and made her own history there. She was Johnno's sister but she had a dominant personality and quickly became an academic and President of the Drama Society. Her most revered scholastic achievements were realized at the University of Cambridge in London where she earned her PhD and returned to lecture here at UWI.

I still see a gentle spirit that calms you at the Mere Sight of her. There is no chance that my rendition of this 5 months old baby could capture her true likeness, just like words will not accurately express the accolades she now deserves. So as I fumbled to render her in my sketch, this caring, loving soul that walks in God's pureness and follows his way; I stumble over superlatives and can't capture the essence that is My Sister.

She has been a great support and is especially caring now during my illness. We live adjacent to each other and share our daily lives. The wall that separates our homes cannot separate our love. I respect her humble humanity enough to not reveal her reserved life and her right of privacy to not intrude. I pray for her continued blessings and that she has a richly rewarding 50th Birthday!

Dr. Alana Ingrid Nicole Johnson is still my baby sister!

http://x.co/66gvG

They want to say I don't care

Last night I laid in bed ready to fall off to sleep and as I promised, I decided to count the many blessings my friends have been to me.

There are so many people that individually showed me exceptional charity and others, who in their normal path of extraordinary care, have blessed me in some way. When you can no longer help yourself and become dependent on others around you, sometimes you feel like a burden and May Shy away from asking for help. My mind is still very fit and my body is too stubborn to obey. It used to be that My Stubbornness worked the other way, I was quick to say no even when my body said yes. In a way, even then my body and mind were in conflict with each other.

The rains come in an unexpected pour and catches me away from shelter. Today, my mind begs my body to run, hurry and get out of the down pour but my mulish body doesn't respond and in seconds I am drenched.

I can see these conflicts between mind and body and it is because I do, I work them against each other. When my body wants to cry out in pain, when the nerves in my hands send signals to my brain with a ghost truck rolling slowly over them, I send messages from my mind, stubborn responses telling the hand, it's MS - Mock Sport. I will pain away whenever I can by being stubborn in my mind and ignoring my body.

I am not sure how effective it is at the neuron levels but I do know that when I sat up in the hospital bed and the tour of doctors peered into my eyes to check my optic nerves, they concluded the same thing. "Given the obvious damage, he is blind in one eye and could barely see from the other." A condition of optic neuritis. Thankfully my mind and body are feuding, each stubborn to the other. I don't see perfectly, but I am not blind in any eye. Maybe my nerves are too frayed for synaptic transmission but an able spirit affords me vison by faith and not by sight.

So, there I laid in bed, already aware of My Short comings but didn't expect this one to plague me at this rested time. I told my mind and my body what was about to happen. I was to think of the people who blessed me in their separate ways and by counting these blessings, I was to fall asleep. It was not to be. My anomic aphasia prevented me from listing my friends. I know all of the treasures they have shown me and felt blessed to have them but my mind was unwilling to conjure their names and I fell asleep with only two name passing my lips. I know the many people out there that I feel blessed to have, even for a brief moment in my life, but it is painful and a miserable feeling not to be able to remember their names.

Some psychiatrists pontificate that the failure to remember names is based on a person's conception of relative importance of the people they forget. I strongly differ and know that people I hold in great esteem can slip away just as easily as passing strangers. When prompted by some incidence, their names can reach the surface but often they have been flooded beneath the vast pleasurable memories etched in my heart.

I may not remember your name initially but I strongly recall our moments together and the blessing I have in you. The physicians were wrong about My Sight and these theorists are wrong about me not caring enough to remember.

I remember you and all you have done to bless my life. I never stopped counting the memories last night and fell asleep with you on my mind

Things will happen

There will be things to happen in life that you will never be able to control or prevent. There will also be things that happened to you in life that will try to shape your will and health and by health I mean all kinds of health; emotional, financial, social, spiritual and physical health. None of us are immune from these things but all of us have a choice in the way we receive them.

I am far from being as Job, "a perfect and an upright man, one that feareth God, and escheweth evil" but I sure intend to be as close to him as I possibly can. His example many centuries ago still speaks to us today.

We all have adversity and troubles but we all have might too and should never forget to lean on its strength. Part of nurturing of this might within us comes from the encouragement we give each other as you have given me. I am Made Stronger because you and others have given a tap on the back of encouragement that says not only do you believe I could but you are contented with what I do.

Cheers my friends

"Sometimes you want to go where everybody knows your name, and they always glad you came."

I was greeted when I arrived by familiar faces and a very recognizable spirit of camaraderie. The evening was going to be a challenge from the moment I agreed to attend. I had not been out at night for over 10 years, save the one time I went to the reunion 5 years ago.

Finding something to wear that wouldn't bring on a seizure was the first obstacle. Then it was timing meals with the dogs and I, to ensure we were all fed, relaxed and ready for the appointed collection time. Everything went perfect, and I was taken to the school and ushered a place to sit after saying a few hellos.

As the time went on I noticed the faces in the Hall were less and less familiar. The older faces I had come to see regularly no longer showed and the reasons were somber. The young faces from years ago had grayed and wrinkled and in many cases had become unrecognizable. And of course, the faces I had never seen but could recognize, their spirit of our hallow walls were obvious and although they never came over and introduced themselves to me where I sat, I felt amongst friends, family, people with whom I was kindred.

If you have read this far then you probably would have been great company listening to me babble about the times I totally enjoyed Combermere, and why it is that I would venture out from my house, me a now clinically recluse, to be there with people I can hardly call by name.

The treat of Chickugunya poses and even greater risk to people with preexisting conditions and is often fatal. My next challenge would therefore be, avoiding a mosquito bite which is now more of a threat than walking into a dark alley. I enjoy what seemed to be a mosquito free night where I sat.

Friends came over to me and shared some time and memories and I want so much to thank them all. I wish it were possible to get up and mingle, to warmly embrace them all, but though the spirit is willing the body is weak and unable.

When I saw the skirts getting shorter as ladies arrived, I knew the time was drawing nearer for the second phase of the night and time for me to leave. My Strict bed time on Fridays is one hour later than other nights and it was already that time. But I didn't need a clock to tell me it was time to go. The music that bellowed the room was creating vibrations on my clothes, tingling my body and tast becoming focal seizures. I know the sensations having experience them so often. I knew I had to make a hasty departure, which for me is a painfully slow walk to most. By the time I saw the same generous faces at admissions, I was already feeling like I was wearing an armor of steel and could only utter quick farewells. We got home safely and after 10 minutes out of the car I was already feeling better.

I express a very special thank you to the President and Executive Committee of the CSOSA for making this a very memorable night which will now be a fantastic memory and a talking piece to some patient and caring ears. I also send a big thank you to the many old scholars who came to sit with me or spend some time and thought nothing of my inability to work the room. Most of all, a great thank you to my friend since primary school, all through school and now 35 and more year after we have left this Waterford academy for making lives and longtime bonds. His modesty does not allow personal accolades but Ralph has shown the trueness of friendship and brotherhood and by our motto Religione, Humanitate, Industria – a true Combermerian.

I feel ashamed to say that the Dale Carnegie course to help me remember names, despite its helpfulness to most others, it did little for me. I still suffer with acute anomic aphasia. In fact, apart from not being able to freely get up and come over to you last night, I was somewhat paralyzed by the inability to remember your name. So sorry! This anomic aphasia seems likely to be a part of me for life and I wish my friends to understand that it does not in any way mean those memories we shared are clouded.

In fact, I seem to hold those memories more vividly than other people and your radiant smile with me is an everlasting picture, clearly before me.

I am sorry to learn you have any condition that will vary from normal health and take away your opportunity to spread that sunshine you always brought with you. Happy though to know you are not daunted by anything. Stay great. Up and On!

It has been 10 years

Hi Karen, thanks for your kind frankness. I was diagnosed with MS 10 years ago and have been learning to adjust to its many faces. They say it affects everyone differently and this seems likely since it is the degradation of one's nervous system, there being millions of nerves, and those affected are random. The most recent episode is with my tactile nerves, the ones responsible for touch. When stimulated consistently they become like needle pricks, tighten the muscles and may induce focal seizures - seizures in the area of agitation. When the hand is affected, I describe it as the "truck" because it feels like a truck is driving over the hand slowly.

But as gory as it Might Seem, MS has made me More Spiritual and I treat the episodes as my body making Mock Sport with Me Since there is no truck.

Hope you get to link up with the old scholars in a meaningful way and that we all can see to the needs of our fellow alma Mater Siblings. Ever upward to the fight!

The Nostalgia was so thick last night we could have sliced it. One of the more touching moments for me was to watch the antics by old scholars that identified them. Facial recognition is out of the question; even if time played no part in distorting their faces, my impaired vision no longer allows. So there I was sitting observing them in conversation, putting names when I could and this one person who was present when you and I came to school, in the More Senior classes, was very familiar but only one name came to mind. He eventually turned and shook my hand as though he recognized me and I said, "Please forgive me, but only Boar Cat comes to mind" His response was something I will always treasure. He told me if I remembered "Boar Cat" then I really know and remember him. He was elated and appeared affectionately moved by so harsh a nickname. The Spirit of Combermere is fantastic and like you, is a great part of me

This is the life

Some years ago I awoke to a new norm. My world was about to change, in fact, it started from the moment I opened my eyes. I took my well-being for granted and expected to be a healthy man as long as I continued to not abuse or use the vices of men.

My biggest flaw was working too many hours in a day and not taking vacations. They called Me Superman and workaholic. I enjoyed my job and found rewards in being of service to the many retail clients. Also, it was a welcomed challenge to ensure my staff felt and did the same.

Some said I was married to the job. If that were true, my morning of change effected a quick divorce after a short separation.

My doctor diagnosed from many tests; including MRIs, CAT Scans, Ultra Sounds, X-Rays, ECGs, EEGs, Lumbar Tap and others, a strange and long name illness, Acute disseminated encephalomyelitis (ADE). It was troubling that I was having the symptoms that suggested this tragic illness but it was treatable and according to the doctor, I could expect to return to good health very shortly. Those were reassuring words as I laid in the hospital bed, hopeful of the things I was yet to achieve. Seemingly improved, they discharged me in about 5 days. Within a week later, I lost sight in one eye. This and other anomalies led to a garrison of tests again.

Only this time it was a year of repeated tests that eventually resulted In the diagnosis of a more familiar illness, one I learned shortly afterwards, few knew enough about. The lifelong and debilitating illness which exists to most as a simple name MS, is a more pervasive and terrifying disease. Multiple Sclerosis can wreak havoc in so many ways, and in every one differently because it is the malfunctioning of nerves which like tissue is throughout the body. There is no way of determining which nerves of the millions will be affected in any MS case. In mine, the eyes, mobility and tactile nerves - those responsible for the touch sensation, were the ones most affected. As a consequence, my vision is impaired, mobility is unsteady, and light, caressing touches are painful.

I lost all perception of color so the flowers in plants disappeared, the sky was always gloomy grey and a look outside, radiant sunlight rendered only shades of black and white. Rainbows no longer existed and people were Mere Shadows in a room. I couldn't see light properly so there were no light bulbs from the ceiling, no street lights and the television was only a grey box of audio.

The slightest breeze knocked me off my feet. Balance was so bad that when an old girlfriend visited and I met her car in the road, I off balanced when she gave me a cake to hold and I dropped it. I was like a child again, but my brain was still an adult. A viable, strong business man who could no longer stand on one foot, or run out of the rain. My physical frustration swiftly got on my emotional nerves. I became short tempered, confused, and irritable; feelings I had long learned to control and for years laid dormant. I was easily moved to tears at the slightest show of humanity

Thankfully, and I truly believe with God's blessings, I got back My Sight. Not the excellent 20/16 they once were but enough that I could enjoy the flowers, the leaves, the birds, butterflies and most importantly, I could see faces again.

That is where you come in, Facebook, my window into life, my opportunity to see you and go where you went through your shares. I may not be able to venture out of my house often but I feel complete when I live through your eyes and bodies. I still don't use obscenities but I learned to read pass them and see how much more there is to people. Their soft sensitive insides beyond crusty exteriors.

On days like today, how generously you stop by to say hi, and leave well wishes for a happy day. I am more pleased to have brief bouts of you now than I was when I could run, drive and dance but didn't fully appreciate you. Yes, I enjoyed those times too but here, now, today I get to see the world through your eyes, enjoy your special occasions. I succeed when you succeed and cry when you do.

I live because you live. I am thankful to all my well-wishers, those whose simple wishes make my day all the more worth living. It was a friendly "Hi" that once led to some of the most rewarding days of my life and it was here on Facebook that it started.

When you think of me, know that I have MS and that it doesn't have me. Know that the MS in my life has given me you and other wonderful memories that I would have missed, married to the job. Know that my MS has made me More Spiritual and that I rejoice in My Saviour. Know that My Salvation is secured and that I use my days More Sensibly and I'm no longer trapped in the Mental Slavery that once overwhelmed me. Although I am here on my own, I am not alone. My Sheikal, actually she is My Sister's, occupies a great deal of my time. This young Akita is now 5 months and no longer needs me in the same way as she did before but she has grown like others, respectful of my illness and supportively at My Side when I go into the front with her.

My friends, I am more grateful for you than I could possibly say, even in this long rant. Thank you for all you do; you make this life worth living!

www.ingramcontent.com/pod-product-compliance
Lightning Source LLC
Chambersburg PA
CBHW020438290526
45785CB00002B/910